MAKING DOWN SYNDROME

MEDICAL ANTHROPOLOGY: HEALTH, INEQUALITY, AND SOCIAL JUSTICE

Series editor: Lenore Manderson

Books in the Medical Anthropology series are concerned with social patterns of and social responses to ill health, disease, and suffering and how social exclusion and social justice shape health and healing outcomes. The series is designed to reflect the diversity of contemporary medical anthropological research and writing and will offer scholars a forum to publish work that showcases the theoretical sophistication, methodological soundness, and ethnographic richness of the field.

Books in the series may include studies on the organization and movement of peoples, technologies, and treatments, how inequalities pattern access to these, and how individuals, communities, and states respond to various assaults on well-being, including from illness, disaster, and violence.

For a complete list of titles in the series, please see the last page of the book.

MAKING DOWN SYNDROME

Motherhood and Kinship Futures in Urban Jordan

CHRISTINE SARGENT

RUTGERS UNIVERSITY PRESS
New Brunswick, Camden, and Newark, New Jersey
London

Rutgers University Press is a department of Rutgers, The State University of New Jersey, one of the leading public research universities in the nation. By publishing worldwide, it furthers the University's mission of dedication to excellence in teaching, scholarship, research, and clinical care.

978-1-9788-4102-4 (cloth)
978-1-9788-4101-7 (paper)
978-1-9788-4103-1 (ebook)

Cataloging-in-publication data is available from the Library of Congress
LCCN 2025019460

A British Cataloging-in-Publication record for this book is available from the British Library.

References to internet websites (URLs) were accurate at the time of writing. Neither the author nor Rutgers University Press is responsible for URLs that may have expired or changed since the manuscript was prepared.

♾ The paper used in this publication meets the requirements of the American National Standard for Information Sciences—Permanence of Paper for Printed Library Materials, ANSI Z39.48-1992.

rutgersuniversitypress.org

CONTENTS

Foreword by Lenore Manderson   vii
Transliteration and Anonymization   xi

1   Down Syndrome and Kinship Futures   1

2   Disability Imaginaries   22

3   Aftershocks   41

4   Ambivalent Interventions   60

5   Getting Stuck   79

6   Aging Uncertainties   97

7   Acceptance   114

     Acknowledgments   121
     Notes   123
     References   141
     Index   167

FOREWORD

LENORE MANDERSON

The Medical Anthropology: Health, Inequality, and Social Justice series is concerned with the diversity of contemporary medical anthropological research and writing. The beauty of ethnography is its capacity through storytelling to make sense of suffering as a social experience and to set it in context. Central to our focus in this series, therefore, is how social structures, political and economic systems, and ideologies shape the likelihood and impact of infections, injuries, bodily ruptures and disease, chronic conditions and disability, treatment and care, and social repair and death.

Health and illness are social facts: the circumstances of maintaining and losing health are always and everywhere shaped by structural, local, and global relations. Social formations and relations, cultures, economies, ecologies and political organizations all shape experiences of illness, disability, and disadvantage. The authors of the monographs in this series are concerned centrally with health and illness, healing practices, and access to care, but in the different volumes, they highlight the importance of such differences in context as expressed and experienced at individual, household, and wider levels. Health risks and the outcomes of social structures and household economies (for example, health systems factors), as well as national and global politics and economics shape people's lives. In their accounts of health, inequality, and social justice, the authors move across social circumstances, health conditions, geography, and their intersections and interactions to demonstrate how individuals, communities, and states manage assaults on people's health and well-being.

As medical anthropologists have long illustrated, the relationships between social context and health status are complex. In addressing these questions, the authors in this series showcase the theoretical sophistication, methodological rigor, and empirical richness of the field while expanding a map of illness, social interaction, and institutional life to illustrate the effects of material conditions and social meanings in troubling and surprising ways. The books reflect medical anthropology as a constantly changing field of scholarship, drawing on research in such diverse contexts as residential and virtual communities, clinics, laboratories, and emergency care and public health settings; with service providers, individual healers, and households; and with social bodies, human bodies, biologies, and biographies. While medical anthropology once concentrated on systems of healing, particular diseases, and embodied experiences, today the field has expanded to include environmental disasters, war, science, technology, faith, gender-based violence, and forced migration. Curiosity about the body and its vicissitudes remains a pivot of our work, but our concerns are with the location of bodies in social life and with how social structures, temporal imperatives, and shifting exigencies shape life courses. This dynamic field reflects the ethics of the discipline to address these pressing issues of our time.

As the subtitle of the series indicates, the books center on social exclusion and inclusion, social justice, and repair. The volumes in this series illustrate multiple ways that globalization and national and local inequalities shape health experiences and outcomes across space, how economic, political, and social inequalities influence the likelihood of poor health and its outcomes in different settings. At the same time, social and economic relations enable the institutionalization of poverty: they produce the unequal conditions of everyday life and work and hence powerfully influence who gets sick and who is most likely to survive. The books challenge readers to reflect on suffering, deficit, and despair within families and communities while they also encourage readers to remain alert to resistance and restitution—to consider how people respond to injustices and evade the fissures that might seem to predetermine their lives.

Christine Sargent brings us to Amman, Jordan, and into the lives of women who have children with Down syndrome. Down syndrome is a genetic condition, not a disease. But its biological origin, of abnormal cell division that results in extra genetic material from chromosome 21, makes it an obvious candidate for medical anthropologists to study, particularly in a series that centers on how inequalities influence health, well-being, futures, and life outcomes. In *Making Down Syndrome: Motherhood and Kinship Futures in Urban Jordan*, we enter the lives primarily of mothers of children with Down syndrome to understand how they work with and against, and imagine, the physical and social limitations of their children as a result of the condition. From their viewpoint we come to appreciate and share the challenges they and their families face in the present and in the conceivable future.

Down syndrome's incidence, worldwide, is around 1 in 1,000 births, including in Jordan. Here, support for families with Down syndrome is primarily provided by community organizations and is largely concentrated in the capital city of Amman. Amman shares with other major centers around the world high levels of care for medical conditions and comprises a well-informed and networked civil society containing allied health professionals committed to early intervention to support children with various conditions in relation to morbidity risk, functional limitations, and capability. Down syndrome has no geography, but location matters as an index of the capacity of families to access such support services and to socialize with other families.

The challenges that trouble women in Amman's families with children with Down syndrome are, to some extent, shared by all families who live in an environment of political volatility, insecurity, and economic precarity. Nearly half of Jordan's population resides in Amman, crowded into the dense inner city and its expanding suburbs. Nearly half of the city's residents are refugees and immigrants, and this number increases if one includes Jordanians of Palestinian descent. Some, for three-quarters of a century, have found refuge in Amman from countries across the region, contributing to a vibrant mix of people from Islam and different Christian sects. Others have newly immigrated either directly from their country of origin and conflict or have arrived as secondary refugees, expelled from their first homes of resettlement. Few refugees are sequestered into camps; rather, immigrants, refugees, and citizens live together across a city that fades from its substantial homes in West Amman into the congested, sometimes neglected tenements of East Amman. Poorer neighborhoods have largely impoverished infrastructure and unreliable public transport, and while in theory the life chances of a child with Down syndrome are stable, the interventions available to parents can shift these chances in predictable ways. For all that is unique to Amman and Jordan, as we learn through Christine Sargent's subtle exploration of class, gender, and location, persistent inequalities within communities override the geopolitical present to influence conceptions of Down syndrome family futures.

Early intervention is promoted to reduce the risk of medical conditions associated with the syndrome, including thyroid dysfunction and congenital heart disease. Speech and language interventions for Down syndrome, introduced from the first year, are designed to address delayed speech and language development and difficulties with articulation, fluency, and intelligibility. Occupational therapy and physical therapy are introduced to enhance motor skills, balance, coordination, and muscle tone to optimize motor development, improve functional abilities, and enhance independence.

As Christine Sargent illustrates, the implications of having a child with Down syndrome are ever present, shaping how mothers envision their children's future in relation to employment, residence, sociality, family making, and long-term care. This informs women's commitment to early intervention and their understanding of its time sensitivity. In one poignant account, Christine describes toddler Shuruq, with her mother, Umm Shuruq, and an older sister, who are eager to learn what to do for Shuruq's physical, speech, and occupational training (*tadrib*) to address potential developmental delays and disability. But Shuruq is frail, recovering from hospitalization for a serious viral infection and complications. The mother is admonished and the family sent home, with a few basic activities and reiteration that the child be allowed to recover and gain strength.

How these women relate to their infants and small children is only the beginning of an evolving relationship over time, as the children age and as they—mothers and children both—struggle to imagine the unfolding future. Infant care everywhere is hard work but arguably unproblematic, likely because care providers—mainly mothers—anticipate and work toward their child's relative independence physically, functionally, and emotionally. But chronic disease, aging, and disability foreshadow the converse, as over time independence decreases, and the need for others' care increases. Early childhood interventions for children with Down syndrome, and for children with other developmental challenges and neurodiversity, moderate this trajectory but do not dilute the ongoing need for care and support.

In elaborating this in Amman, Christine brings us into women's everyday lives, their understandings of their children, and their continued concerns. Few mothers regarded marriage as an option for their children, and women with sons in particular saw marriage as added work and responsibility for them and others in the family. Who would take care of them, Umm Sami asked, elaborating on her vehement rejection of her husband's relatively liberal and idealized wish that Sami enjoy the love, care, and companionship of an adult relationship. "If he gets married to another girl like him," Umm Sami continued, "there will be two people who need to be taken care of."

Most women worried about their continuing capacity to undertake the physical work of care and who would take it up when they were no longer around or no longer capable. Umm Fadi, for example, pondered over the future of Fadi, her teenage son, who would soon be too old to participate in educational and social programs and who needed support for his health. She insisted she would keep Fadi at home while she was alive. She had other children, but who might step up to the task of care was, she emphasized, "their choice." The question was therefore unresolved. Age, life stage, gender, and the constraints of Down syndrome on autonomy left young adults and their families "stuck" between roles and life stages.

Making Down Syndrome brings us into the lives of an extraordinary community of feisty women determined to ensure their children's capabilities; they celebrate their children's skills and sociability. At the heart of this is the women's commitment to family and their understanding that their child with Down syndrome is a gift from God and that by honoring this gift, they carry the responsibility and the privilege of care. For women in Amman, at least, their assumed and accepted role as the primary caregivers and their perception of their children's continued dependence on them shape how they manage, what they do, and what they worry about, on a continuing and evolving basis.

TRANSLITERATION
AND ANONYMIZATION

I have transliterated Arabic terms using a modified version of guidelines provided by the *International Journal of Middle East Studies*. Most of my interlocutors spoke a dialect of urban Arabic that would be locally recognized as Palestinian Jordanian, and I have tried to retain phonetic and stylistic elements of their speech. This means that some transliterations diverge from what would be expected in Modern Standard Arabic (Fusha). Given the recognizability of *umm* (mother) to Arabic speakers, I chose not to transliterate its more common dialectical pronunciation, *imm*. For the sake of readability, and to minimize distraction for non-Arabic speakers, I have omitted long vowels, diacritics, and phonetic transliterations of "sun" and "moon" letters. Errors of transliteration and translation are entirely my own.

I provide pseudonyms for all persons and institutions who participated directly in my research. Norms around this practice continue to shift, reflecting concerns with intellectual theft masked as anonymization. While closely following these conversations, I believe that pseudonyms best honor the dense and sometimes complicated relational networks that my participants belonged to, both personally and professionally. In places where I mention scholars, activists, or self-advocates by name, I do so in reference to published works and media or public appearances.

.

MAKING DOWN SYNDROME

1 · DOWN SYNDROME AND KINSHIP FUTURES

"The most important thing."

On a sunny spring day in 2014, I found myself in a small public garden tucked beside one of Amman's major north–south arteries. A rarity in the sprawling capital, the surprisingly quiet oasis hosted a seasonal weekly farmers market. Not to be confused with Amman's bustling downtown shops (*al-balad*) or popular Friday souq (*souq al-jum'a*), the market's organizers sought to create a calm, contained atmosphere where young adults with intellectual disabilities and their families could socialize while supporting small businesses.[1] Having connected through my nascent research on Down syndrome, I showed up hoping to be helpful, and a coordinator stationed me alongside a fellow volunteer selling small cups of Arabic coffee.

After I initiated the proper protocol of salutations and introductions, the older man warmly invited me to call him Abu Yehya—literally, "father of Yehya," a teknonym I used in my daily interactions with parents and preserve throughout this text.[2] As we promoted our thermos of coffee, Abu Yehya kept a steady eye on his son Yehya, who was then in his early twenties. Yehya basked in the market's pleasant buzz and wove his way through the sea of tables, chairs, and booths stationed along the edges of the park's grassy knoll. Making new friends and greeting familiar faces, he faithfully circled back to provide his watchful father with a steady stream of updates. As I observed Yehya's continuous loops, I found their father-son resemblance striking, both in build and even more so gregarious affect.

When I explained that I was a doctoral student studying families' experiences with Down syndrome, Abu Yehya began nodding enthusiastically and exclaimed in heavily accented English, "Ask me anything!" Then, without pausing to see whether I had anything specific to ask, he switched back to Arabic and continued: "The most important thing ... The fundamental thing is that the family accepts them [the child with Down syndrome]. In Arab society, often if a woman gives birth to a sick child, the husband leaves. Not me! The most important thing is the mother and father, then the family—siblings! My siblings have daughters, so they didn't want Yehya to be seen, because they want their girls to get married." To stress this point, he pantomimed locking a door and throwing away the key. "This is how Arab society thinks. If someone is disabled, the family is disabled." Returning to his list, he added additional components and ticked his fingers off one by one, which culminated with him waving an outstretched palm in the air. "The mother, the father, the family, neighbors, society. And another thing," he added. "There's no government support."

Abu Yehya placed kin at the center of a disability world (Ginsburg and Rapp 2013, 2024) where acceptance, alongside a sense of disability-as-hazard, flowed between people and through relationships rather than attaching to bounded body-selves. "My siblings have daughters, so they didn't want Yehya to be seen, because they want their girls to get married." The moment marked one of many where people positioned disability not first or foremost as identity, nor as an individual experience, but rather as an interdependency lived between kin.[3] I eventually visited Abu Yehya and his wife, Umm Yehya ("mother of Yehya"), at their home in northwestern Amman, where we spent the afternoon discussing their nearly three decades as a "Down syndrome family." This phrase, which I have borrowed from my interlocutors, stretches Down syndrome beyond the boundaries of a discrete bodymind (Price 2015; Schalk 2018). In doing so, it speaks to two of my main goals in this book: centering kin relations as a primary locus for *making Down syndrome* and highlighting how Down syndrome transforms *kinship futures*.

As they answered my questions and steered our conversation in new directions, Umm and Abu Yehya crisscrossed between present, future, and near and distant past. Memories of diagnostic shock gave way to contemplations of looming financial uncertainties. Reminiscing on celebrations held to honor their newborn son blurred into worries over current health ailments and anticipatory frailties. These twists of time recurred throughout my fieldwork, with parental projections into the future—and past—eclipsing our shared present, and they led me to carefully contemplate Down syndrome's temporalities alongside its evident relationality. Neither of Yehya's parents minimized that sickness and disability could introduce tensions between kin and community. But Abu Yehya proudly identified as an exception to the apocryphal man who abandoned his wife and child. And Umm Yehya rejected the inevitability of flighty husbands or cruel relatives, even as she confirmed the pervasiveness of these disappointments.

Both parents described acceptance (*taqabbul*)—an emic category that reappeared over the course of my research—as a lifelong process of learning to resist the injurious ideas, beliefs, and practices that people without Down syndrome, themselves included, attached to Down syndrome. Acceptance meant envisioning and enabling a future where Yehya could grow up and grow old beside his family, and that future required them to remake their existing world. Eventually, I came to see acceptance as a mode of "being-with" (Al-Mohammad 2010) and a mode of anticipation. Acceptance incorporated Down syndrome into the relationally imagined and enacted life course that I refer to throughout this book as a *kinship future*. Kinship futures, in turn, *make* Down syndrome's bodily, social, and political possibilities cohere by cultivating—or constricting—networks of care.

KINSHIP FUTURES

When I started my research, I asked everyone I met: If I want to understand Down syndrome in Jordan, to whom do I need to talk? Mothers were considered such an obvious answer that I instead received advice about *which* mothers to talk to—and whom to avoid. Mothers drove interpersonal and societal quests for acceptance, even as they remained uncertain about what acceptance demanded from them or how to demand it from others. That I met Umm Yehya through her husband proved highly atypical in my fieldwork, a point I will return to in my later discussion of care. Yet it served as an important reminder that mothers rarely operated alone, even if they sometimes felt acutely lonely. Abu Yehya placed mothers first in his list of "most important things," a role they occupy in this ethnography as well. This is because mothers operated as key nodes in the relational networks of care that make Down syndrome.

Mothers of younger children often advised me not to rely on older women. Their experiences had been so traumatizing (or so the argument went) and so little once existed in terms of services and support that they could not comprehend the world inhabited by Down syndrome families in the mid-2010s. Mothers of older children, however, and many of the teachers and therapists I met thought that I should concentrate my research on aging families. Childhood with Down syndrome was not "the problem," they told me. Growing up and growing older, however, introduced intractable challenges for individuals and family units. These competing strands of advice helped me to appreciate that while changing social conditions make Down syndrome at different historical moments, what Down syndrome *is*, and what its acceptance entails, depends on how individuals and families age together and apart.

This is why conversations about Down syndrome seemed to precipitate time travel, especially for mothers. A newborn raised questions about marriages that would not happen for decades; a first grader generated anxieties about stable employment and retirement savings; a teenager's romantic longings led to reflections on old age and mortality. As one woman explained while worrying about her eldest son's performance in school and her youngest daughter's struggle to access schooling with Down syndrome, "Parents *here* depend on their children for the future. I encourage my son to excel not just for his own personal growth but also for my sake, for my own well-being when I get older. I will depend on him." In emphasizing "here," she implicitly contrasted Jordan with "the West" (al-Gharb), a place widely associated with familial estrangement, social anomie, and moral breakdown. It also revealed a future imagined and built through expectations attached to noninterchangeable relations between kin. These included (but were not limited to) the following: what sons owe to mothers, when daughters will marry and shift their focus to husbands and children, and how a shared sense of accountability before God stretches moral economies of care beyond the boundaries of death.

"Domains of kinship and reproduction," write the anthropologists Rayna Rapp and Faye Ginsburg, are "key social sites at which many disabilities are initially assigned cultural meaning" (2001, 536). While far from the postindustrial and (questionably) democratically governed Global North hubs of disability studies knowledge production, Jordan's local realities intensified the political and economic stakes of Ginsburg and Rapp's argument. Alongside and even beyond questions of meaning, I focus on making Down syndrome through kinship futures. By this I mean the hopes, fears, and claims that wove Jordanian futures through the warp and weft of kin relations. Would the presence of visible disability damage a cousin's marriage prospects? Would an adult son or daughter accept responsibility for housing a sibling who could not support themself? Would parents outlive a child with a compromised immune system, and what did it mean to hope for such an outcome?

Accepting Down syndrome into kinship futures looped back to make Down syndrome's daily, embodied realities, while having a child with Down syndrome transformed the horizons of imaginable kinship futures. In thinking about kinship futures, I draw on the disability and crip studies insight that ideologies of temporality, and especially futurity, constrain disabled lives and politics in the present.[4] More specifically, I engage Alison Kafer's (2013) articulation of "crip futures," a term that expresses her longing for imagined futures that respect disabled peoples' existence and affirm disability's value. Crip futures challenge the hegemony of futures imagined through a prism of "curative violence" (Kim 2017), wherein disability's absence or eradication signals societal progress.

While crip and kinship futures overlap, the latter preserves the distinctly kin-oriented futures that my interlocutors imagined.[5] They also reveal a paradox at the heart of making Down syndrome: that disability can forge new and even radical paths for claiming kin and creating community while also reproducing hierarchical and normative social structures. In Jordan the latter hinge on heteronormative marriages, patrilineal reckonings of family and belonging, and inegalitarian, patriarchal economies of care that transform but also endure under the pressures of structural adjustment. And while geopolitics may recede from the affective thrum of everyday life, shared borders with Occupied Palestine, Israel, Syria, Iraq, and Saudi Arabia seep into kinship futures and how they make—and unmake and remake—Down syndrome over time.

MAKING DOWN SYNDROME

Shortly after Yehya was born, his doctor alerted his parents to differences in their son's eyes, mouth, tongue, hands, and palm lines, identifying markers of Down syndrome that are often visible at birth, especially to a trained medical professional. He then informed them that their son would be "slightly r-tarded" (*'andu shway takhalluf*) and "have some disabilities" (*wa shway i'aqat*).[6] Umm Yehya was less concerned with these blunt pronouncements and more so with whether she would be able to hold, kiss, hug, and play with her son. Much to her relief, the doctor confirmed that Yehya would certainly be capable of such things. Years before Yehya was born, his parents watched one of their older children succumb to fatal illness, a heartbreak that formatted their reception of their youngest son's Down syndrome. While the doctor marked various aspects of Yehya's bodymind as exceptional, his parents deemed those same traits unremarkable. Would Yehya be affectionate, social, and engaged—Would he *survive*?

According to the medical model of disability that Yehya's parents encountered in the hospital, Down syndrome is "the most common genomic disorder of intellectual disability worldwide" (Antonarakis et al. 2020, 1). Down syndrome results from trisomy (triplication) in human chromosome 21. The errors in cell division responsible for creating extra chromosomal material occur during the development of the sperm or the egg, and trisomy does not pass from parent to child in all but a minority of cases.[7] Individuals with trisomy in chromosome 21 experience distinctive phenotypic features, developmental delay, and intellectual impairment, and they are at higher risk for congenital heart defects.[8] They are also susceptible to a variety of health conditions across the lifespan, especially early-onset Alzheimer's disease (Cipriani et al. 2018).

How does acceptance contribute to making Down syndrome? A brief glance at the past century offers some insights. In the mid-1900s, life expectancy for a child with Down syndrome in economically advanced countries hovered between ten and twelve years. As of the mid-2020s, this number stands at sixty years of age (Bittles and Glasson 2004; Carr and Collins 2018; Glasson et al. 2002). Better health interventions have played a role in this shift, but they are reflections of broader cultural transformations (Kaposy 2023; Piepmeier 2012; Thomas 2021, 2024). As recently as the 1980s, physicians in the United States—with backing from state supreme courts—supported parents who chose to decline lifesaving surgeries for infants with Down syndrome (Fost 2020). The presence of Down syndrome negated what would, for a nondisabled child, be considered unethical or even criminal medical neglect. And today, despite the increasing visibility and flourishing of people with Down syndrome, noninvasive prenatal technologies position the condition as a bioethical litmus test in debates about disability and selective reproduction, at least in Global North contexts (Agarwal et al. 2013; Estreich 2016; Kaposy 2018; Löwy 2017; Piepmeier 2021; Rapp 1999; Thomas 2017, 2024).

Ultimately, the unitary label of "Down syndrome" belies the diversity and spectrum of impairment experienced by people living with variations in chromosome 21. It also has little to say about the relationships with kin, community, and God that my interlocutors emphasized in their accounts of what is now widely recognized as *mutalazimat Down* (see chapter 2). Drawing from medical anthropology and disability studies, I follow how relationships, practices, and institutions make Down syndrome through embodied practices of care. Making captures the interface of how clinical classifications "make up people" and how disability gets done (Hacking 1999; Mol 2002). The first considers diagnostic labels and the "looping effects" by which actors and institutions take up and take on the possibilities that these labels afford (Hacking 2004). The latter pushes ethnographers to move beyond meaning and pay closer attention to how bodily realities emerge through practice.[9] Focusing only on perspectives and interpretations would leave Down syndrome untouched as "a single passive object in the middle" (Mol 2001, 5). *Making* widens the scope of analysis. It allows me to ask how practices of care intersect with skin, muscle, bone, pathogens, policies, and events that make up lives and worlds to make Down syndrome's (many) realities.

Embodied and social experiences gathered under the mantle of Down syndrome increasingly "hang together somehow" (Mol 2002, 5), as evidenced by transnational community building and advocacy networks. Yet they do so unevenly across divergent political and cultural contexts. Given the open wounds of occupation and war that reverberate across much of Southwest Asia and North Africa (SWANA), academic, policy, and development initiatives often concentrate on disability resulting from armed conflict and other cascading forms of postcolonial violence (Aciksoz 2019; Dewachi 2015; Puar 2014; Rubaii 2020).[10] Yet neither violence nor inequality directly result in Down syndrome, and most of the families in this book lived at further (but never total) remove from the urgency of crisis. Many forces contributed to making Down syndrome in Jordan: chromosomes, emotions, muscles, therapeutics, pedagogies, laws, and human rights conventions, to name a few. But I focus most closely on relationships—especially those between mothers and their children.

MOTHERS, MARRIAGE, AND CARE

"The mother is the foundation" (Al-umm hiyya al-asas). Time and again, mothers, special educators, and therapists encouraged each other with this phrase when strategizing about advocacy or reminding each other of their obligations and responsibilities. On the one hand, it attested to the power they felt they could—and must—wield to change themselves and their society. But it also gestured to continuities between colonial and postindependence regimes of governance that assign women overwhelming responsibility for realizing culturally, nationally, and religiously inflected visions of progress (Abu-Lughod 1998; Ahmed 1992; Deeb 2006; Kandiyoti 1991). The mothers who take center stage in this book belong to Jordan's highly educated female population, which nevertheless makes up less than 15 percent of the workforce, a "gendered paradox" that continues to frustrate development orthodoxy (Adely 2012a). In a relatively short time span, these women have gained expanded access to social networks, educational opportunities, and labor markets beyond kin and home, even as they never fully depart from the gravitational pull of the latter.

Disability ethnography across divergent contexts has shown that intimacies of patriarchy and ableism link mothers and disabled children through structures and ideologies of care (Blum 2015, 201; Fietz 2020a, 2020b; Friedner 2022b; Landsman 2009; Thomas 2021; Williamson 2024; Williamson et al. 2023; for a focus on fathers, see Jackson 2021). A notoriously expansive and slippery term, I understand "care" to include the complex and often grueling labor of social reproduction (Buch 2015), as well as emergent processes of coming-to-matter (Stevenson 2014). Synonymous with neither love nor empathy, care can reproduce personal and systemic forms of inequality and even amount to violence (Aulino 2019; Buch 2018; Mattingly 2014a; Glenn 2010). In Jordan, class-privileged women partake in an "international division of reproductive labor" (Parreñas 2000) by hiring paid domestic workers from Africa and Asia to execute the daily tasks of social reproduction—cooking, cleaning, childcare, and, increasingly, eldercare (Frantz 2008, 2010, 2013; Gordon 2020).[11] But this practical outsourcing remains financially out of reach for most, and it has not unsettled a pervasive narrative that assigns care to the domains of kinship and motherhood.

In Jordan, the status of "mother" remains closely linked to that of "wife." Actual relationships fail, stall, and unravel, but marriage remains a crucial arbiter of kin ties. While patrilineal descent conveys powerful social recognition, lawful marriage mediates the legitimacy of paternity (Hughes 2021). The designation of "orphan," for example, can denote children with no living parents, those with unknown parentage, and those born out of wedlock (Engelke 2019). Legally excluded from patrilineal belonging, orphans experience lifelong negative social, legal, and financial consequences (Farahat and Cheney 2015; IRCKHF 2017). Marriage and descent acquire further force through Jordan's Nationality Law, which prohibits women married to non-Jordanian men from passing their citizenship to their husbands or children (Amawi 2000).[12] The Personal Status Law (PSL) that governs marriage and related matters further codifies patriarchal norms and patrilineal authority into law through the provision of guardianship (*wilaya*).[13] This legal structure assigns a male guardian decision-making authority in matters of schooling, medical treatment, and travel for minors and unmarried women under forty (Almala 2014; HRW 2023).[14]

As a simultaneously social, legal, and religious institution, marriage inflects the making of Down syndrome by structuring how people negotiate constraints on care and contemplate their interwoven kinship futures.[15] A rise in the median age at first marriage (22.5 years of age for women and 27.5 for men), shifting betrothal practices, and increasing judicial scrutiny of marriage contracts have contributed to a widespread sense that marriage is in "crisis" locally and across the region (Hasso 2011; Hughes 2021).[16] Debates surrounding the extent and origins of this crisis attest to how tightly marriage regulates interlocking structures of gender, sexuality, and kinship.[17] From a macro perspective, Jordan's changing marital trends coincide with other significant demographic transitions, including shrinking households, decreasing fertility rates, population aging, and longer life expectancies (Alhalaseh 2019; Puschmann and Matthijs 2012). Together, they are transforming how families provide care and anticipate future demands.

Spending most of my time with women helped me connect what might otherwise appear as unrelated facets of making Down syndrome in Jordan: an acute sense of "responsibility" assigned to mothers and a pointed concern about daughters with disabled siblings. Kinship futures linked mothers and daughters through a modality akin to that of *straight time*, or "the convergence of the normative directionality of rehabilitation and 'cure' with the aspirational futurities of heteronormativity" (Wool 2021, 289). In Jordan, straight time narrows more decisively into *marriage time*. Women think *care-fully* about the future because gendered inequalities and asymmetrical interdependencies of care span a lifetime. They are perpetuated by social norms, reinforced by law, and exacerbated by difficult economic and political conditions. The woman who explained to me that she will rely on her son when she gets older was then caring for her own aging, chronically ill mother-in-law while managing her son's academic struggles and advocating for her daughter. She found herself faced with the unenviable task of monitoring her mother-in-law's diet, which led to recurring conflicts over the contents of their refrigerator. Her situation was far from unique. Many women live near or co-reside with their mothers-in-law while trying to care for their own aging parents and parenting their own children.

Gender shaped how people understood their care prerogatives as spouses and kin, but it did not overdetermine the complexities of their actual relationships. Umm Yehya, for example, struggled with chronic health issues and limited mobility, so she could not accompany Yehya to the market on the day I first met her husband. Abu Yehya, retired, mobile, and full of energy, eagerly volunteered to accompany his son, giving Yehya an opportunity to socialize and his wife time to rest. In confronting responsibilities of caregiving and disability, their family met shifting constraints with creativity (Dokumacı 2023). Mothers were not the only caregivers within families, and care was by no means limited to kinship. How families dealt with everyday contingencies of care, which often intensified in the presence of disability, attested to their shared broader circumstances and the singularity of their unique relationships and personalities. But my ethnography nevertheless pivots around mothers because they proved so critical to organizing and distributing care across and beyond family networks.

PROXIMITY TO DISABILITY IN A DIVIDED CITY

Shadowing a group of women from West Amman while they delivered Ramadan meals in Jabal Ahmar, one of the city's poorest eastern neighborhoods, I watched a recipient cautiously approach a volunteer named Umm Khaled.[18] "Can I ask you something?" the older woman queried hesitantly. Originally from rural Palestine, she had recently relocated to Jordan with her two intellectually disabled adult sons. Previously, her sons had rarely left their family's home, but a new neighbor convinced her to enroll them in a crafts program run by a local nongovernmental organization (NGO) partnering with the West Amman group for their Ramadan initiative. "Please don't get offended," she prefaced. "Forgive me if the question is rude." Umm Khaled warmly reassured the older woman not to worry. When we later debriefed this exchange, she admitted how, in the moment, she could not fathom what was about to happen. "I thought she was going to ask if I'm in Daesh [ISIS]!" Umm Khaled joked.[19]

The older woman looked at Umm Khaled, took a deep breath, and continued. "Do *you* really have a disabled child? Like *me*?" Umm Khaled's eyes widened in surprise. "Yes, truly! My son Khaled has both intellectual and physical disabilities." As she scrolled through her phone to pick her favorite photos of Khaled, another member of our delegation explained that she, too, had a disabled son. The NGO employee accompanying us on the delivery route shared that she had a brother who was physically and intellectually disabled, although he had recently passed away. The older woman appeared stunned, quietly absorbing these displays of affirmation while also managing to murmur "Allah yarhamu" (God rest his soul) for the employee's recently departed brother. Moments when women discovered shared "proximity to disability" (Rutherford 2020) could be transformative. But they also illuminated how serendipity and systemic inequality made disability disparate, in part by reproducing women's responsibilities as caregivers, advocates, managers, and peacemakers who had vastly uneven resources available to manage these undertakings.

This unevenness manifested in the city itself as much as through encounters between the women who lived and navigated its contradictions. Nearly half of Jordan's population resides in the governorate of Amman, which includes the city's densely inhabited core and its expanding suburban perimeters. But a sense of Amman as "contingency" bubbles through depictions of this com-paratively young city (Shami 2007, 209), with its fragmentation manifesting in discursive and material divisions between West and East (El Zein 2020; Hourani and Kanna 2014; MacDougall 2019; McLaughlin-Alcock 2020; Parker 2009). The West Amman neighborhoods where more affluent Ammanis like Umm Khaled lived are home to Jordan's government ministries and foreign embassies; glittering (and heavily securitized) shopping malls; five-star hotels; and cafés, bars, and gyms whose aesthetics are decidedly vague. Gender segre-gation is uncommon (although some spaces offer women or family-only rooms or floors), and a variety of eastern and western aesthetics comfortably coexist, including a plurality of Islamically inflected sartorial practices (Abbas 2015). Moving from west to east, the tenfold population increase that Jordan experienced in a mere fifty-five years becomes visible and palpable (DOS 2015).

West Amman is defined by at least some degree of spaciousness—between buildings and bodies—while some of East Amman's poor and working-class neighborhoods boast population densities among the highest in the world (Ababsa 2013b). Local butcher shops, spice vendors, and fruit and vegetable stands serve clientele who complete shopping trips on foot, although encroaching supermarket chains are a cause for concern among small business owners, while the "Credit Is Forbidden" signs posted in every West Amman *dukkan* (corner store) disappear. Public spaces are decidedly masculine, and most women wear abayas, jilbabs (dress-like overcoats that come in a variety of colors and styles), or thobes (a dress with wide sleeves and a tapered waist) adorned with embroi-dery patterns (*tatreez*) that communicate cultural patrimony and typically Pales-tinian origins. Some of the city's oldest Christian communities also call East Amman home, and one can find Armenian Catholic, Anglican, Syriac Orthodox, Nazarene, and Greek Catholic churches located within the span of a few blocks.

When I traveled to East Amman by taxi, drivers would double- or triple-check my destination, a process complicated by the fact that I rarely knew where I was going. Nor were street names particularly helpful; excluding Amman's major east–west and north–south arteries, landmarks serve as more reliable locating devices. (The ability to "pin" one's location and send coordinates via WhatsApp, as well as the arrival of Uber, have ameliorated these struggles for locals and visitors alike.) Whenever my friend Reem collected me from a major bakery at the crossroads of East and West Amman to bring me to her home, my generally foreign appearance and messy bun of uncovered hair attracted con-fused stares from fellow motorists stuck in traffic, much to the amusement of Reem and her children. In West Amman, beyond the stares that all women who occupy public space learn to navigate, my presence and appearance were unre-markable. I read as another tourist, student, or employee at one of the many humanitarian organizations, embassies, and consulates that cluster around spe-cific traffic circles in the city's western "half."

Despite glaring divisions in wealth, theorizing class in Amman can neverthe-less prove challenging (Nasser-Eddin 2019). Traditional data points like "home-ownership" may be misleading, given that "half the residents of Amman's poorest informal settlements are [considered] homeowners" (Ababsa 2013c). Yet other dimensions of class can be gleaned from how people talk, move, shop, dress, and navigate space. These are the embodied and felt dimensions of privilege and inequality that Pierre Bourdieu (1977) refers to as habitus and that I attend to more closely throughout this book. At the same time, I remain wary of how scru-tiny over Muslim women's dress may tell us less about their class and position-ality than about the sartorial fixations of primarily Western and non-Muslim audiences.

Like the many residents who traverse East and West Amman for school and work (Schwedler 2010), Down syndrome also crosses the city's partitions of class, ethnicity, race, and citizenship. In the chapters to come, I concentrate on moments when women found each other through proximity to disability, which often also brought their different conceivable kinship futures into sharper relief. These moments did not always entail dramatic acts of recognition across difference, nor did existing social fault lines magically dissolve to make way for harmonious solidarities. But given the lack of integrated or geographi-cally embedded systems for building disability networks at that time, Amman's disability-focused spaces fostered connections between an unusual cross sec-tion of the city's inhabitants and even those from surrounding governorates.

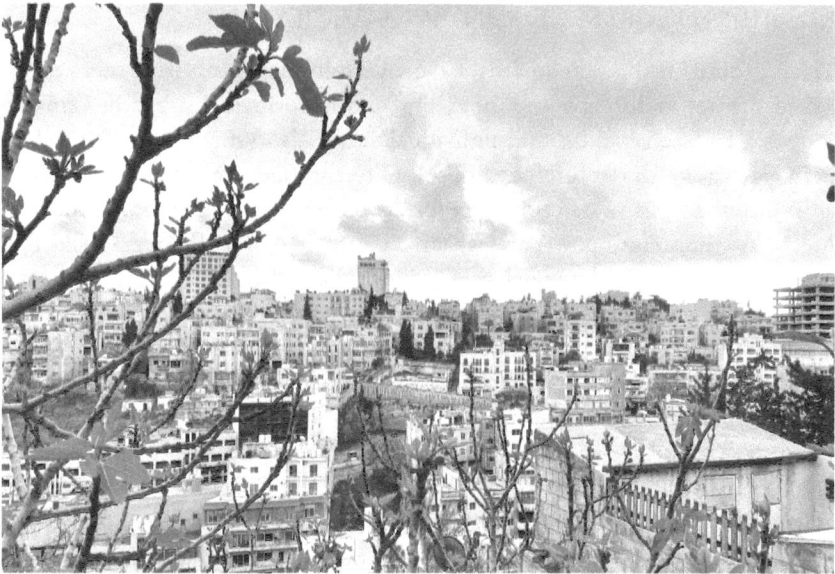

FIGURE 1. A view from Jabal Weibdeh across to Jabal Amman (two of West Amman's oldest neighborhoods). Photo by author.

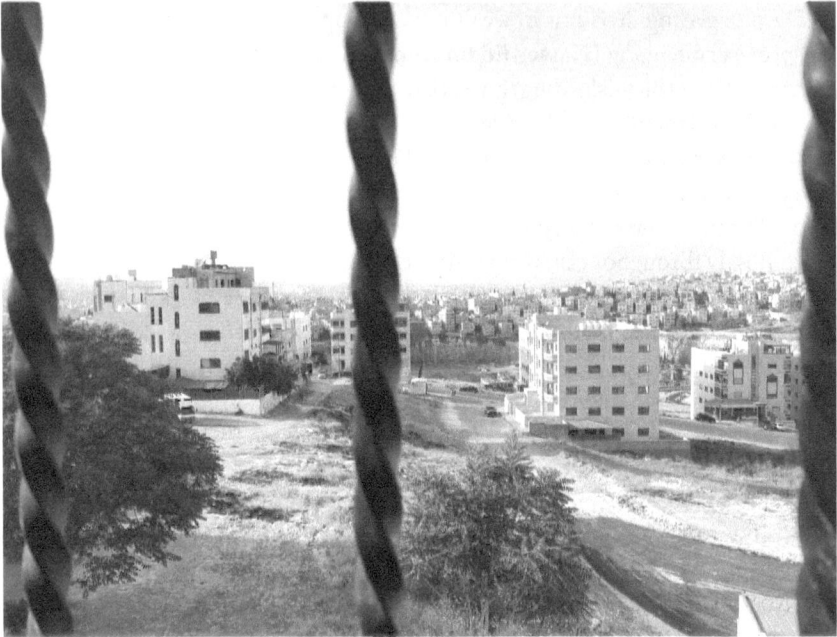

FIGURE 2. A view from the balcony in a rapidly expanding neighborhood of East Amman. Photo by author.

KINSHIP FUTURES, COLONIAL LEGACIES

Tracing social life through the lens of Down syndrome departs from more established themes in Jordanian ethnography and historiography, but the kinship futures I trace on familial and individual scales also refract Jordan's modern political history. Under four centuries of Ottoman rule, the region once known as Transjordan was valued primarily for its location on the pilgrimage route to Mecca. Administrative power and wealth concentrated in northern cities like Salt and Irbid, where wealthy merchant families from Syria and Palestine built networks of commerce and kinship across highly permeable political boundaries. But during the Great Arab Revolt (1916–1918), Jordan's geographic and political centers of power reassembled around the Hashemites, a powerful family with roots in the Hejaz (contemporary Saudi Arabia).

Spurred in part by British promises to support a unified Arab state, the Hashemites led an uprising that successfully expelled the Ottomans from the Hejaz and Transjordan. Yet in the aftermath of World War I, the League of Nations brought its own strategy of rule to fruition, dividing the region into colonial mandates. The British government considered Transjordan a critical buffer between Iraq and Palestine, so it created the Emirate of Transjordan in 1921 and installed Abdullah I as its leader. With Amman designated as the newly Hashemite center of power (Méouchy et al. 2013), Emir Abdullah began stitching together what would become the monarchy's core support base: Circassian farmers, Transjordanian tribes, and Christian merchant families.[20] Today, Jordan's constitution protects the Hashemites' authority to rule in perpetuity, a claim they ground in their role as sharifs (custodians) of Islam's holy sites, their descent from the same lineage as that of the Prophet Muhammad, and their role in the 1916 revolt (Katz 1995; Layne 1994).

Two years after gaining its independence in 1946, Jordan's political and economic trajectories were permanently altered by the establishment of the state of Israel. In 1947 the United Nations (U.N.) General Assembly decided to partition mandate Palestine into Jewish and Arab states, precipitating a displacement crisis whose devastation continues into the present.[21] The period of violent dispossession known throughout Arabic-speaking countries and the global Palestinian diaspora as Al-Nakba, or the "Catastrophe," thrust nearly 1 million Palestinians into refugeehood as they fled widespread ethnic cleansing campaigns helmed by Israeli militias (Allan 2021; Khalidi 2020; Pappe 2007). A minority of displaced Palestinians remained inside the 1948 borders of Israel, but most fled to Jordan and Lebanon, with smaller numbers settling in Syria and Iraq.

This early influx of Palestinian refugee communities rewrote Jordan's nascent politics of class and ethnicity, which were further transformed by the Six-Day War in 1967, when Israel occupied the West Bank and Gaza, and the Gulf War (1990–1991), when Kuwait and other Gulf states expelled their Palestinian residents (Al-Nakib 2014; Mason 2009). In the aftermath of these traumatic ruptures, hundreds of thousands of Palestinian refugees made their way to Jordan. And while Amman's oldest camps now blend into the fabric of the cities surrounding them, they bear signs of material and infrastructural neglect (Ababsa 2013a; Achilli 2014, 2015).[22] Schools and health clinics attest to the enduring presence of the U.N. Relief and Works Agency (UNRWA), although seventy-six years of displacement have strained the organization to a breaking point (Feldman 2017; Gabiam 2012, 2016; Hanafi et al. 2014).[23]

These recurring upheavals have made Jordan an instructive site for analyzing contradictions and limitations of humanitarian governance, with much of this scholarship focused on Palestinian refugees—both those with Jordanian citizenship and those who remain stateless (Feldman 2018; Pérez 2018; 2021).[24] Long-simmering and sometimes violent conflict between Jordanians of "East Bank" origins and those of "West Bank" Palestinian descent, which graft onto fault lines of economic opportunity and inequality, are central to local formations of ethnicity, class, and race, as well as the Hashemites' political calculations and constraints (Alon 2009; Fischbach 2000; Massad 2001; Shryock 1997). My fieldwork, however, coincided with a dramatic transformation in Jordan's humanitarian landscape.

The iconic tents (now trailers) of the Zaatari camp, built in 2012 to shelter refugees from Syria's civil war in a remote northeastern corner of the Zarqa governorate, generated massive investments of aid and surveillance infrastructures (Awamleh and Dorai 2023; Dalal 2020; Musmar 2020). Jordanians and foreigners often assumed that I would focus my research on the Syrian crisis. The praise I received for not doing so gestured to widespread resentment toward the estimated 1 million refugees who now comprise 7 percent of Jordan's population.[25] For many Jordanians of Palestinian descent, who represent the country's presumed but intentionally uncounted majority, the international response to Syria betrayed long-standing indifference toward Palestinian suffering, while those of Jordanian descent lamented that the country again found itself buckling under a human catastrophe not of its making.

My interlocutors identified as Jordanian (both "Jordanian Jordanian" and "Jordanian of Palestinian origin"), Palestinian from the Occupied Territory, Syrian, and Iraqi; some were emigrants residing in Arab Gulf countries, Europe, Canada, or the United States who returned for extended visits, especially during holidays and the summer months of June and July. Some were official refugees, while others were displaced but managed their presumably permanent relocation through Jordan's system of residency visas. Syria's war and the long shadow cast by the 2003 U.S. invasion of Iraq surfaced repeatedly in their stories.[26] As women observed and compared experiences of mothering children with Down syndrome, they integrated these salient axes of privilege and marginalization into their analyses.

Women of Palestinian descent often described Jordanian negotiations with disability as complicated by the more tribal dynamics of their kin networks.[27] Kurds and Circassians, both Jordanian and Syrian in nationality, distinguished themselves from Arabs and Palestinians by self-identifying as less "conservative" in religious and gender norms. My "Jordanian Jordanian" interlocutors were no less forthcoming, cataloging the mentalities and temperaments they associated with different segments of Jordan's multiethnic and increasingly multiracial society while offering especially pointed commentary on the "Palestinian psyche." Almost all my interlocutors were Muslim, but the time I spent living with a Christian family in the governorate of Madaba (south of Amman) granted me insights into how members of Jordan's religious minority (approximately 2% of the population) navigate tensions of solidarity and difference.

Women also stressed categories that united them across difference, which included being Arab (or non-Arab), Muslim, and Middle Eastern. And through their identities as mothers, they imagined and claimed affinity with Down syndrome families around the world. Observing and connecting across countries, continents, and languages, these local and virtual encounters amplified how shared and radically dissimilar circumstances made multiple realities of Down syndrome possible.[28] They also made sense of my presence through these same circuits of connection and distance.

RAPPORT AND POSITIONALITY

"Multi-sited" sounds more elegant than "frantically and dizzyingly peripatetic," but I would opt for the latter in describing fieldwork (Marcus 1995). My personal sense of chaos and dislocation, however, seemed to match that of some mothers as they "pioneered" new sites and networks for making Down syndrome (Rapp 1999). While imagined futures stayed anchored in relations and spaces of kinship, the pragmatics of making Down syndrome compelled mothers—and me—to depart from the domestic and domestic-adjacent spaces well represented in SWANA anthropology (Abu-Lughod 1986; Hoodfar 1997; Jansen 1987; Meneley 1996).

In the nearly two years I spent in Amman between 2013 and 2015, I relied on tactics that paralleled those of my interlocutors. This included touring special education and residential centers, meeting special educators, therapists, and activists who invited me to visit their practices and organizations, and attending awareness-raising events and free medical screening days marketed toward disabled children and their families. Very little of this occurred systematically. I met families through other families; I joined WhatsApp groups; I kept a close watch on public Facebook events because invitations begot more invitations. And while I did not directly engage with Jordan's Higher Council for the Rights of Persons with Disabilities (HCD; see chapter 2), I crossed paths with some employees more informally, and I benefited immensely from their research and publication activities.

Across these different strands of fieldwork, I strove to cultivate what literary- and disability studies scholar Julie Avril Minich describes as "disability studies as methodology" (2016). This methodological orientation resists a biomedically driven gaze and shifts attention to "the social norms that define particular attributes as impairments, as well as the social conditions that concentrate stigmatized attributes in particular populations" (Minich 2016). This meant that I met and spent time with non–Down syndrome families whose children received generalized designations of intellectual and developmental disability, as well as more specific diagnoses of cerebral palsy, autism, or multiple disabling conditions. These labels facilitated shared experiences of stigma and structured similar pathways for seeking services, but they also revealed divergent social codings of impairment, which shaped how families confronted and navigated the question of acceptance.

I spent a considerable amount of time at an organization that I call the Al-Nur Society, which focused on providing early intervention services and advocating for disabled children's right to access public education (among other issues). Beyond Al-Nur, I created a separate web of connections through my friendship with Reem, a special educator I met through a mutual colleague. Reem and I bonded over similar "ethnographic sensibilities" toward the world around us (McGranahan 2018), intrigued by questions of disability, culture, and kinship and notwithstanding our otherwise dissimilar professional and personal lives. Having then completed a master's degree in special education, Reem supplemented her teaching and administrative career by providing lessons—early intervention, speech therapy, literacy, and homework support—to local children. She allowed me to station myself in the salon of her family's East Amman apartment, where I met her clients and neighbors as they arrived for sessions or passed by simply to visit, and she invited me to accompany her on professional and personal trips to meet clients and kin.

Despite the different worlds I inhabited across the city, many of my interlocutors knew each other, or at least knew of each other, either through Al-Nur, or because their children attended one of the well-established special education centers located in West Amman, or because they participated in social outings facilitated by civic and nonprofit organizations. They were usually friendly, but they were not necessarily friends. Some identified as belonging to a Down syndrome "community" or even a broader "family." Others did not, despite the pervasiveness of kinship terms in Down syndrome spaces and events. Al-Nur provided a critical hub for my research and relationships, but I do not focus extensively on the organization out of respect for their operations and the many changes in policies, staff, and circumstances that have occurred since my fieldwork.

As I crisscrossed Amman and its ever-extending suburban parameters, I built a city rich with disability spaces and energies, and I started seeing disability everywhere. Trendy restaurants in West Amman integrated workers with Down syndrome into the waitstaff. The public bus route I took to visit my former host on the outskirts of Madaba consistently included a group of deaf people signing to each other. And a cadre of high-profile disabled politicians and activists leveraged social media to remind people that disability has always been part of Jordan's social fabric. But my perspective clashed strongly with my interlocutors' sense that disability was "hidden" and needed to be brought into view. My independent and mobile lifestyle undoubtedly contributed to our conflicting experiences. The inaccessibility and unaffordability of transportation in Amman (and Jordan more broadly) created barriers to moving around the city, especially for women (Abu Moghli et al. 2018; Aloul et al. 2018).[29] Yet these opposing perceptions also reflected our different relationships to Jordan's overarching disability imaginary, which I detail in chapter 2.

The rootlessness that led me to see disability "everywhere" shaped my access and engagement in other ways. My lack of attachments—as a foreigner and a non-Arab, non-Muslim woman, unmarried but of marriageable age and devoid of recognizable kin networks—generated concern and even pity (but also admiration, especially among younger Jordanians). It marked me as a particular kind of stranger. On the one hand, how well could anyone expect to know me, or I them, in the absence of legible social coordinates? Others appreciated my distance from their densely knit social networks; they did not need to worry about complications arising from unexpected and undesired ties to their kin or community. "Home" could be ambivalent, and many women erred on the side of caution in considering the impact that my presence might have on their lives. They valued organizations like Al-Nur for combining aspects of domestic-like intimacy with time and space away from spouses, in-laws, parents, and (sometimes) even children. Much of my data come from observations and conversations in these more liminal spaces, neither wholly domestic nor completely removed from home and family, where women cultivated new knowledge, intimacies, and distances (Deeb 2006; Ossman 2002; Tobin 2016).

Regardless of where and how I met research participants, my American-ness invited conversation and occasionally caustic commentary, especially given the unpopular impact of U.S. pressure on Jordan during that point in its campaign against the Islamic State. As one of the perennially highest recipients of U.S. foreign aid, the Hashemites' capacity (or willingness) to depart from U.S.-driven policy priorities remains limited, and the government has embraced economic and foreign relations policies that have proven immensely unpopular with the Jordanian people. The United States' unwavering support for Israel, despite expanding illegal settlements in the West Bank and the terror inflicted on Gaza's already immobilized and suffering population with Operation Protective Edge (2014), was never far from my Palestinian interlocutors' minds.

Many foreign ethnographers in Jordan find themselves the subject of jokes—cloaking cautious, earnest probing—about their potential employment by intelligence agencies (Hughes 2019; Martínez 2022). Others report less pointed but no less serious inquiries as to their *actual* research interests (Mason 2021). I did not feel as closely scrutinized in this regard (at least overtly), perhaps because many people considered disability a plausible research "problem" and a well-established humanitarian and development issue. Legibility, however, did not exempt me from accountability. When I forgot the Arabic term for "punishment" ('iqab) and stared blankly at my closest interlocutor, Umm Farha, while frantically flipping through my mental flash cards, she briefly switched to English and delivered a lesson in vocabulary retention. "Punishment, Christine! Punishment! America punishes the whole world, and you can't even remember the word!" Her indignation combined the teasing and sharp-tongued social commentary that characterize our relationship to this day, and I have never since forgotten the meaning of 'iqab.

My citizenship afforded me the privilege of crossing borders with ease, which some families hoped I could leverage in support of their quests to secure visas for themselves or their family members. It also sparked recitations of personal and diasporic geographies, as people listed the cities where family members had emigrated to or were resettled as formal refugees, in many cases as a direct or indirect result of U.S. military action. Alongside these always-present dynamics of nationality, race, religion, and gender, many women positioned me as a student beyond the relatively inscrutable field of anthropology. They sought to guide me through lessons about marriage and motherhood—and makeup—while politely seeking reassurance that I planned to move forward with these critical (and in my case, delayed) stages of life. That I was neither the mother of a disabled child nor a mother at all intensified this "younger and possibly wayward sister" dynamic with those I became closest to, while others regarded me with relative indifference or even suspicion.

VOICE, ETHICS, AND ACCESS

The social networks that I created while circulating through and beyond Amman did not consist exclusively of mothers and other kin. In addition to special educators and rehabilitative therapists, I spent considerable time with children and adults with Down syndrome. Given their importance to my fieldwork, I want to further address why the latter do not figure into the text as *direct* interlocutors. The space I give to mothers reflects my methodological and theoretical orientations. I wanted to understand how people responded to the embodied differences that Down syndrome precipitates, and how this specific label was gaining legibility, so I focused on the parents—and especially the mothers—who play powerful roles in these processes.[30] This in no way diminishes the importance of other makers of Down syndrome, not the least of which includes people with Down syndrome themselves.

Scholars in disability studies and disability anthropology have strongly objected to the overrepresentation of parents and mothers in disability-focused research (Kasnitz 2020; McGuire 2016; Thomas 2024). This is a concern I share and continue to grapple with in my work. A major criticism is that centering parents displaces disabled people's own narratives, further subjugating an already marginalized population. On this point I want to be clear: Mothers, fathers, siblings, and other caregivers are not proxies for the narratives and experiences of people with Down syndrome. But the cumulative actions of these differently—and unequally—positioned actors form the broader tapestry of kinship futures that make Down syndrome's everyday realities.

This leads me to a second criticism, which is that working with parents can perpetuate bias by depicting them as benevolent heroes. Parents are capable of and often responsible for inflicting violence against their children. While this was not something I witnessed firsthand, ample evidence from Jordan and elsewhere confirms this bitter reality, especially for disabled children. Even activism driven by nondisabled parents, which often plays a critical role in disability rights movements, may sharply contradict disabled people's own agendas and desires (Carey et al. 2020). I approached mothers and children as a nexus for hierarchical relations that connect kin through care (Gammeltoft 2008), but I do not view this nexus through rose-colored glasses. In chapters 5 and 6, especially, I detail how interdependencies of care created conflicts between mothers and children as pressures of aging shifted family members' priorities and capacities. Yet it would be equally inaccurate to depict their relationships solely in terms of oppression. Love, laughter, and wonderment coexisted alongside frustration, disappointment, and even despair. Parenthood, regardless of a child's disability status, can profoundly challenge and change one's sense of self and the world.

Finally, concerns about the capacity to consent can create obstacles for research participants with intellectual and cognitive impairments. Anthropologists, among others, have been at the forefront of developing participatory methodologies that challenge ableist institutional barriers and the reductive equation of disability with vulnerability (Cascio and Racine 2019; Eli-Long and Quinn 2022; Patterson and Block 2019). But beyond the purview of institutional review boards, ethnographers remain accountable to the ethical demands set by our interlocutors. I approached participant recruitment as a collective and relational endeavor rather than as interactions between autonomous individuals; this meant navigating relationships between parents and children. Given the latter's significant lack of autonomy in their daily lives, and regardless of age, I felt uncertain about my ability to guarantee their privacy or confidentiality.[31] Families did not require a panel of scholars to validate their assessments of who counted as vulnerable, and they maintained their own expectations about what appropriate responses to vulnerability entailed.

My focus on mothers emerged as I navigated these considerations at a particular juncture in my life. I made decisions based on my positionality and personality (the existence of which anthropologists seem hesitant to acknowledge), which in turn had an impact on my data collection and analyses. This does not negate the collective nature of making Down syndrome. Nor should it be understood as an uncritical celebration of motherhood or kinship more broadly. Yet dismissing motherhood or deeming it unworthy of study seems equally misguided, especially given the mother-blame discourses that appear throughout disability histories (Blum 2015; Ryan and Runswick-Cole 2008; Runswick-Cole and Ryan 2019; Sousa 2011). People with Down syndrome know no other life or sense of self than the lives they live and the selves they become *with* Down syndrome. Their choices and opportunities, however, are deeply entwined with how kin and strangers make this label (or others) accrue meaning and materiality. Mothers operated as arbiters and sometime-disrupters of the norms and relations "that define particular attributes as impairments" (Minich 2016). These norms and relations created possibility and vulnerability for those with Down syndrome—and those without. What, then, is this book about? It is an ethnography of kinship, motherhood, and Down syndrome and the ambivalent, sometimes painful interdependencies that connect all three.

OVERVIEW OF THE BOOK

The arc of kinship futures structures the chapters to come, which (after chapter 2) travel through specific stations along a normative "life course." I do this to highlight the tensions between this ideal model, where life proceeds along a linear pathway, and the unpredictable discrepancies that can decouple aging from socially defined markers of "age" (Laz 1998). Despite its distance from reality, this model maintained a powerful grip on making Down syndrome. It shaped how specific impairments became disabling at different points in time, even as lived experiences with disability also led families to imagine new ways of aging and flourishing.

In chapter 2, "Disability Imaginaries," I offer a contemporary history of disability in Jordan. While Jordan is widely regarded as a regional leader in disability rights, I use the concept of *disability imaginaries* to flag how the category of disability refracted colonial and Orientalist discourses about Jordanian "culture." These manifested in debates about hiding and inclusion, which are twin poles in local disability imaginaries. To illustrate how they operated in practice, I turn to the high-priority issue of inclusive education. Despite Jordan's progressive laws and policies, families navigating the realities of actual schools brought their own concerns to bear on the possible meanings and manifestations of inclusion.

Chapter 3, "Aftershocks," tracks the imaginative and practical labor that mothers performed to make Down syndrome in the earliest stages of life. I focus on the shock (*sadma*) that followed a child's diagnosis and threatened to disrupt relationships between spouses and kin. To contextualize this early and often intense sense of hazard, I consider how kinship operates as a diagnostic technology alongside the advent of more recent biogenetic tools. This meant that a child born with a noninherited condition could still raise fears about family lineage and perceptions of marriageability. Under these circumstances, scientific ambiguity and patriarchal authority colluded to position women and children as exceedingly vulnerable to marginalization.

In chapter 4, "Ambivalent Interventions," I examine the impact of Jordan's expanding early intervention services on childhood disability and motherhood. The ambivalence of these early "interventions" shows how therapeutic programs positioned both women and children as interdependent agents of change and objects of scrutiny. The ethnographic material focuses on formal and informal curriculums of "habilitative care" (Williamson 2024), which became sites for enacting and contesting the boundaries of "normal" bodyminds and of good motherhood.

Chapter 5, "Getting Stuck," focuses on how embodied transitions of adolescence precipitated parental preoccupations with "What comes next?" Between childhood and adulthood, intersecting norms of age, gender, and sexuality assigned the threat of "embodied asynchrony" (Kafer 2013, 48) to the bodyminds of young people with Down syndrome and other intellectual disabilities. This perception of misalignment created starkly gendered implications. While young women's fertility emerged as a problem to control, young men's desires became a problem to manage. Rather than experiencing adolescence as a liminal stage, young people—and their families—became increasingly "stuck."

Chapter 6, "Aging Uncertainties," broadens considerations of embodied asynchrony to consider how aging engendered relational and spatial disjunctures. Mirroring chapter 3's focus on marriage, I shift the generational focus to consider what happens as young people with Down syndrome attempted to access key normative pathways to adulthood: marriage and employment. Drawing primarily on conversations with mothers of adult sons, I highlight how marriage—and its absence—relationally mediated access to housing and capital. Some mothers contemplated possibilities for cohabitation and care beyond the domains of lineal or affinal kin, but the absence of alternatives meant that siblingship assumed an increasingly important role in enacting kinship futures over time.

To conclude, I reflect on the turbulent years that have followed since I conducted my primary fieldwork, and I return to the question of acceptance. The kinship futures described in this book reflect the exigencies and possibilities of a specific moment—the mid- to late 2010s—before the COVID-19 pandemic. As the world settles into an uneasy postpandemic normal, other regional (and global) crises now impinge on disabled lives and the making of Down syndrome in Jordan and beyond. These acute—and long-simmering—calamities will continue to set the malleability and even viability of kinship futures in the decades to come.

2 · DISABILITY IMAGINARIES

"Where are people with disabilities in our society?"

In the summer of 2014, I spent several days at the Al-Nur Society observing a training program open to anyone interested in learning basic principles of early intervention. An umbrella term, "early intervention" covers a range of services and supports for babies and young children with developmental delays or disabilities and their families. In addition to introducing the foundations of a program called Portage (the focus of chapter 4), the training organized guest lectures on special topics, including a session on disability "rights and awareness" (*huquq wa taw'iyya*). The presentation was led by Layan, a human rights expert who had decades of experience working with the bilateral and international development organizations that target Jordan's most vulnerable communities, which include poor rural families and urban-dwelling refugees from Palestine, Syria, Iraq, Yemen, Sudan, and Somalia.

To start her talk, Layan presented the audience—primarily of mothers of young children with Down syndrome—with a prompt. "Where are people with disabilities in our society?" (Wayn al-ashkhas dhowwi al-i'aqa fi mujtama'na?). With a striking degree of consensus, the group replied almost in unison, "They're hidden!" (Mukhabi'in). Layan nodded her head and repeated the word "hidden" for emphasis. She then asked *why* families hid people with disabilities, which generated a variety of responses:

— "fear of behavior" (*khowf min al-suluk*)
— "daughters" (*binathum*)
— "a culture of shame" (*thaqafat al-'ayb*)[1]

The lone husband attending the training alongside his wife then suggested that Islam could contend with this misguided practice, and several women vigorously nodded their heads in agreement. The importance that Layan and the group attached to delineating the real cause(s) of hiding, and their desire to refute its potential misinterpretation (a concern perhaps heightened by my presence), spoke to the cultural dynamics of Jordan's disability politics—and of researching disability in Jordan—that I address in this chapter.

While most of this book focuses on everyday encounters and embodied practices that make Down syndrome over a familial life course, here I zoom out to situate Jordan's recent history of defining and legislating disability. These efforts are key to understanding the vocabulary and grammar of what I refer to as Jordan's *disability imaginaries*. Anthropologists have used "the imaginary" to capture how diverse projects of power/ knowledge (Foucault 1980)—such as medicine (Good 2007), pharmaceuticals (Jenkins 2010), demography (Aulino 2017), prenatal diagnostic technologies (Gammeltoft 2014b)—infuse constructions of self, place, and possibility. Unlike states of "debility" that either belong to the broader human condition or reflect unique signatures of state-sponsored violence (Livingston 2005; Puar 2014), disability imaginaries are tethered to the modern, biopolitical category of disability (Stiker 1999).[2]

Simultaneously intimate and public, local and global, a disability imaginary constrains and enables the work that disability does in any particular corner of the world. Jordanian disability imaginaries remain steeped in narratives about the country as "behind" or "backward," which facilitates a "cultural symbolization" of disability that pits the West as a "heaven for disabled people" against the "hell" of the Global South (Kim 2011, 103; see also Grech and Soldatic 2016; Hartblay 2017; Nguyen 2023).[3] This symbolization occurred through the prism of what anthropologist Mayssoun Sukarieh describes as "culturalism" (2012, 2016), an interpretive framework that "has become hegemonic in shaping interpretations of the Arab world, not just among Western commentators but many Arab elites as well. According to this analysis, there is something fundamentally wrong with 'Arab culture,' a fatal flaw that is holding the region back" (Sukarieh 2012, 119). While changing laws and policies work to reconfigure Jordan's empirical realities of disability, they often do so while reinforcing a broader imaginary in which pathologies of "culture" get blamed for ableism and inaccessibility.

At the same time, dichotomies between the (Global) North and South, or East and West, risk flattening the capaciousness of Jordan's disability imaginaries and oversimplifying the fractal politics of culture and class that sustain them. Activists, government officials, and staff of international nongovernmental organizations (NGOs), many of whom were considered elite by virtue of family lineage or class and educational backgrounds, often identified "beliefs" about disability as a major obstacle to the country's progressive policies. Yet the families I met, fewer of whom would be considered part of this elite, *also* reinforced the terms of this imaginary. They accused elites—and each other—of backwardness and ignorance. This intricate geography of power enabled dissimilar parties to seize a shared language of culturalism-as-critique and direct it toward their desired targets.

In the next section, I examine the central role that hiding played in sustaining local disability imaginaries. As a manifestation of everything "wrong" with disability in Jordan, and everything wrong with Jordan itself, hiding became a local and *cultural* phenomenon that scripted disability into competing claims about backwardness and "modern-ness" (Deeb 2006). The ideal of "inclusion," which stands in opposition to hiding, underwrites many of the laws and policies discussed in this chapter. This is especially true in the realm of education, where inclusive education has become a priority for the Jordanian government and a lynchpin of global disability rights movements. Competing framings of inclusive education can reveal how disability imaginaries operate in practice. Families often hesitated to support inclusive education initiatives. Some questioned whether inclusion represented a "best practice" and for whom; others articulated alternative versions of inclusion that prioritized home and family over school and its questionable relationship to the labor market. Their cautious engagements with inclusion illuminate both the theoretical and methodological "problems" related to hiding and their impact on researching and making Down syndrome.

HIDING AS MYTH AND REALITY

The image of a locked door with a disabled person hidden behind it circulated widely among the Jordanians, immigrants, refugees, and expatriates with whom I discussed my research. When I first started drafting funding proposals for this project as a graduate student, I received warnings from Western-based academics, humanitarians, and development professionals that disability would be extremely challenging to research anywhere in Southwest Asia and North Africa (SWANA) because disability—and disabled people—remained overwhelmingly hidden. As a stranger and a foreigner (and worse, an American), I would struggle to broach such a taboo topic. I also encountered versions of this warning in Jordan, with specialists and advocates bracing me for families' unwillingness to participate and the likely demise of my project. None of these cautionary tales emerged from nowhere, but they reinforced an imaginary that obscures disability's lived complexities through a suspiciously familiar narrative about Arab and Muslim conservatism, seclusion, and culture. And they did not match what was happening on the ground.

In 2012, journalist Hanan Khandagji went undercover as a trainee at several Amman centers (*marakez*; sing. *markez*) for disabled children, which provide segregated educational programming, therapeutic and rehabilitative services, and, in some cases, residential accommodations. Most disabled children in Jordan who attend centers do so as day students, if they participate in programming outside the home at all, and only a minority attend inclusive public or private schools alongside their nondisabled peers. Khandagji documented widespread abuse against students and residents at these centers, most of whom were either Jordanian or citizens of Gulf countries. In collaboration with Arab Reporters for Investigative Journalism, BBC Arabic featured Khandagji's footage in an exposé titled *Behind Walls of Silence* (*Khalaf jidran al-samt*).[4] The film generated significant media coverage and public outrage. In the aftermath, King Abdullah II himself appointed a task force to address the ensuing scandal, which culminated in the arraignment of several administrators on charges of torture and neglect (Hauswedell 2013).

Hiding occupies a powerful place in disability politics and culture because it testifies to the isolation and marginalization that disabled people face around the world. But it also risks collapsing dissimilar historical conditions and social logics into a misleadingly uniform description. "The myth of the hidden disabled," warned the anthropologist Benedicte Ingstad some thirty years ago (Ingstad and Whyte 1995, 246), reflected the tendency of human rights and development initiatives to focus on "attitudes and beliefs" as the primary hurdles facing disabled people in the Global South. Overemphasizing the obstacles posed by mentalities (or "culture") ignores how basic struggles for survival inform disability experience for much of the world's population, especially where support beyond kin collectives is limited or practically absent. It also flattens distinctions between different forms and logics of confinement. In Jordan, as in many places, family collectives and domestic spaces serve as the primary—if not sole—sites of care for disabled children and adults.[5] Accordingly, the "Walls of Silence" that people associated most closely with disability were those of the family home.

Hiding became an enduring but paradoxical thread during my fieldwork, discursively omnipresent while empirically elusive. At least one dimension of this puzzle can be attributed to sampling bias. The women I met sought out services and community. They were willing—even if reluctantly—to enter spaces that centered disability needs and identity (to varying degrees). Families who secluded or denied the presence of a disabled member remained largely out of my orbit. In some cases, however, I met families whose lackluster participation in early intervention or educational programming stemmed from personal or financial hardship that engulfed the entire household rather than reflecting disability-specific discrimination. Hiding definitely obscures more complex realities, but I do not suggest that it can be reduced to a "myth" or "misunderstanding." Throughout my research, people shared their own disturbing encounters with hiding, telling me about obstinate parents who refused to let a disabled relative leave the house and about families that effectively abandoned someone to a residential center. One father recalled his horror when he realized that his neighbor's intellectually disabled daughter wore diapers not because she was incontinent but because her family deemed her incapable of learning, so they never attempted toilet training.

If hiding once "made sense," however, as an acceptable way to protect kin collectives from the potential loss of reputation incurred by disability, this logic no longer cohered by the mid-2010s. Instead, hiding evoked condemnation and confusion, becoming a vehicle for people from widely divergent sectors of society to try and make sense of the vulnerability and violence that disabled Jordanians experienced. Rather than encounter an impossible taboo, I found families navigating dynamic and rapidly changing social and therapeutic landscapes. And far from being perceived as scandalous or insensitive, my questions felt relevant or, at the very least, pragmatically unavoidable. Our conversations became a chance to compare notes and share our respective analyses of Jordan's progress in the realms of disability law and policy, which many interlocutors nevertheless decried as *hiber 'ala waraq* (ink on paper) or *haki fadi* (nonsense, literally, "empty talk").[6] The activists, lawyers, and humanitarians working to translate these gains into practice resented such commentary, viewing it as evidence of Jordan's failure to establish a "culture of rights" among its citizens. Yet I came to see these dismissals of their work as evidence of how families live in the gaps between laws and their implementation, between discourses of rights and the hard truths of social inequality.

Over the past three decades, Jordanians have experienced declining standards of living and widening economic disparities, largely due to World Bank and International Monetary Fund structural adjustment programs (first introduced in 1988) and the government's enthusiastic embrace of further neoliberal reforms (Ababneh 2018; Baylouny 2010; Hourani 2014; Martínez 2022; Yom 2015). As the educated and underemployed population assesses painfully obvious gaps between human rights discourses and the austerity measures that constrain imaginable kinship futures, patience for the former has faltered and waned. And while its autocratic monarchy renders neither citizenship nor liberal and democratic ideals meaningless, Jordan's citizen-oriented politics materialize in conjunction with other axes of power and systems of patronage. The latter, channeled through extended family lineages, tribal networks, diasporic connections, and politicized ethnic affiliations, often prove more reliable for ensuring security and survival. This broader political landscape informed everyday encounters with the identity and rights-based disability frameworks that did not translate smoothly or wholesale into Jordanian contexts.

Nevertheless, diverse and even antagonistically positioned actors across Jordan's social and political landscape recognized disability as a category of international importance—and scrutiny. The "problem" of hiding refracted the moral stakes of disability encounters, which I experienced throughout my research and in writing for primarily Western-based audiences. On the one hand, hiding constitutes a human rights violation that has been well-documented in Jordan and around the world, the persistence of which my interlocutors themselves confirmed.[7] But accusations about hiding highlight how (disability) rights discourses can reinforce colonial and Orientalist tropes that underwrite Jordanian class politics and overdetermine how people live, represent, and imagine disability's realities. These tensions formed the core of Jordanian disability imaginaries, suffusing the choices families made about education and care, the standards by which they were judged, and how they judged others in turn. Next, I unpack some of the key mechanisms for making disability legible through data, definitions, language, and law. This plurality of knowledge forms converged to reinforce the broader terms of Jordanian disability imaginaries.

MAKING DISABILITY

Data. In the fall of 2013, the Washington Group on Disability Statistics (WG) convened in Amman for its Thirteenth Annual Meeting. Established in 2001 under the auspices of the United Nations (U.N.) Statistical Commission City Group, the WG "promotes and coordinates international cooperation in the area of health statistics focusing on the development of disability measures suitable for census and national surveys. The major objective . . . is to provide information on disability that is comparable throughout the world" (2024). Hosted by Jordan's Higher Council for the Affairs of Persons with Disabilities (now the Higher Council for the *Rights* of Persons with Disabilities) and the Department of Statistics, the WG aided Jordan's 2015 Population and Housing Census, a massive and notably high-tech undertaking supported by a bevy of international donors.

The census included a modified version of the disability-specific module known as the Washington Group Short Set (WGSS), which aims to standardize disability data by asking about "degrees of capacity" across six functional domains: vision, hearing, mobility, cognition, self-care, and communication. Foregrounding the question of "function" shifts data collection away from screening protocols and survey instruments that rely on the term "disability," an approach that nevertheless remains common across the SWANA region (ESCWA 2018a). Jordan's 2004 census, for example, utilized a self-identification approach, with census takers asking heads of household, "Do you/does someone in your family have a disability?" The resulting 1.2 percent prevalence rate (Mont 2007, 8) fell staggeringly short of the World Health Organization's estimated global disability prevalence rate of 16 percent (WHO 2022).[8]

The WGSS reflects a global desire for high-quality, quantitative disability data, and its function-oriented questions attempt to address the instability and divergent connotations of the term "disability." Yet the very need for the WGSS gestures to intransigent conceptual challenges. WG guidelines advise countries to calculate their national rate of disability prevalence by combining the responses of "a lot of difficulty" and "cannot do [it] at all." In Jordan, however, this would result in the still questionable prevalence rate of 2.7 percent

(ESCWA 2018a, 14). Current publications, however, typically report Jordan's national disability rate as 11.4 percent, which means that the government includes the response of "some difficulty" in its overall estimates. The discrepancy between these two calculations attests to the inevitable reality that "subjective" interpretation and assessment cannot be extricated from disability data collection or analysis (see Schneider 2009 for a critical assessment of WG methodology).[9]

That Jordan hosted the WG's 2013 meeting points to how some disability imaginaries celebrate Jordan's progressive government while lamenting its recalcitrant citizenry. In his oft cited paper on disability rights in Jordan, for example, the political scientist Kenneth Rutherford describes the kingdom "a pioneering leader of the Arab World" (2007). He attributes Jordan's excellence to three major factors: "an enlightened royal family, a national tradition of openness and generosity, and one of the best educational systems in the Middle East" (Rutherford 2007, 3). The elevated position of Jordan's enlightened royals indicates their central (albeit contested) role in constructions of Jordanian nationalism and in perceptions by foreign and especially Western nations (Nanes 2010; Shryock 2000) that regard the regime as an ally to be supported at all costs, including that of genuine democratic reform (Ryan and Schwedler 2004; Ryan 2011). "The national tradition of openness" that Rutherford later elaborates does not center core values celebrated by Jordanians, such as hospitality, but instead highlights the Kingdom's receptiveness to "foreign" ideas and influences (like disability rights). The article succinctly communicates an imaginary where cosmopolitan Hashemites appear at the vanguard while their challenging constituencies fail to realize the promise of modern laws and policies due to cultural attachments and beliefs.

Definitions. My desire to understand Jordan's "disability worlds" brought me through a wormhole to Washington. This felt especially ironic given that the United States remains among the small minority of U.N. member countries that have signed *but not ratified* the U.N. Convention on the Persons with Disabilities (CRPD). As a clear testament to its global support, the convention acquired more signatories on its opening day in March 2007 than any other convention in U.N. history. Poorer countries spearheaded the convention's coordination and drafting efforts because they recognized the importance of having a mechanism to prioritize disability issues in development policies and funding streams (Meekosha and Soldatic 2011). But like other rights conventions built around a singular figure—human, woman, child—the universalizing category of disability continues to struggle in its encounters with "local (moral) worlds" (Kleinman 1992, 1998; Yang et al. 2007). Consequently, members' hopes of crafting "culture-free" visions of human flourishing and social justice became strained during the actual process of drafting the convention (Ghaly 2019; Kanter 2007).

The CRPD inevitably relies on sociolinguistic categories to map the contours of (disabled) bodies, minds, and persons. The preamble describes disability as "an evolving concept" that results from "the interaction between persons with impairments and attitudinal and environmental barriers that hinders their full and effective participation in society on an equal basis with others" (United Nations 2006a, 1). Article 1 elaborates further, defining persons with disabilities as "those who have long-term physical, mental, intellectual or sensory impairments which in interaction with various barriers may hinder their full and effective participation in society on an equal basis with others" (United Nations 2006a, 4). These wide-ranging categories of "physical, mental, intellectual or sensory" entail philosophical, religious, medical, and popular genealogies that intertwine and unravel over time. The historicity of disability terminology and the shifting cultural sensibilities it reveals can be gleaned from the CRPD's official Arabic translation of "impairments" as *'ahat*. This term gestures to the palimpsest of meanings onto which "disability" has been superimposed (United Nations 2006, ar.).[10]

Historians of disability in the SWANA region consider *'ahat* to be the historical predecessor to the modern Arabic term for disability, *al-i'aqa*. The latter stems from the root verb *'aqa*, which builds off core meanings of "to hinder or prevent."[11] Most literally translated as "blights," *'ahat* carried wider meanings and implications than the contemporary concepts of disability or impairment. According to the medieval Islamic historian Kristina Richardson, *'aha* (sing.) connoted "a mark that spoils the presumed wholeness of a thing" (2012, 5). While some *'ahat* severely limited an individual's status and degree of social inclusion, others did not become disabling.[12] Although Jordanian disability imaginaries position disability on a developmentalist trajectory from hiding to visibility, the Ottoman historian Sara Scalenghe has argued that, at least in the archives, "people with impairments of the body and of the mind are everywhere" (2014, 3). Yet she has also noted that impairments associated with "the mind" appeared to be the most subjected to discrimination and social exclusion, as evidenced by extensive legal and philosophical deliberations about capacity and accountability.[13]

Ethnographically, this older lexicon has largely receded from circulation.[14] Jordan's Law No. 20 of 2017 on the Rights of Persons with Disabilities and its older Law No. 30 of 2007 (now repealed) both translate impairments as *qusur*, although each iteration of the law maps a different corresponding topography. Government institutions and documents make a concerted effort to exclusively use the terms "disability" and "people with disabilities" (*ashkhas* [*min*] *dhowwi al-i'aqa*), with the Arabic rendering of "person-first" terminology predominating in legal and activist spheres. The phrase "special needs" (*al-ihtiyajat al-khassa*) also remains common despite activist efforts to generate a shift toward disability-centered language. More recently, Arab Gulf countries like the United Arab Emirates have begun promoting the phrase *ashab al-himam*, or "people of determination," an increasingly popular but unofficial alternative to "disabled" or "with disabilities" (Department of Social Affairs UAE, 2025). Clearly, disability language—in Jordan and elsewhere—continues to evolve and change.

Language. Many of the parents in my research focused their energies on one language issue: replacing the colloquial term *mongholi* with *mutilazamat Down* or *Down* (*sindrom*). *Mongholi,* which most Jordanians consider an offensive slur, belongs to trisomy 21's unevenly excavated global history (Chen 2023; Pearson 2023; Wright 2011).[15] When British physician John Langdon Down published "An Ethnic Classification of Idiots" in the 1866 *London Hospital Clinical Report,* he was intrigued by the scientific debate of his day: the unity or diversity of the human species. Down argued that the existence of "a Mongolian type of idiocy," in which the "child of Europeans" could "degenerate" into a Mongol, supported arguments for the oneness of the species (Down 1866, 696). Given its origins, opposition to this terminology gained momentum by the mid-twentieth century, and a 1961 statement coauthored by nineteen prominent genetic scientists in *The Lancet* urged medical and scientific communities to find replacements for "mongolian idiocy," "mongolism," "mongoloid," and related labels (Rodríguez-Hernández and Montoya 2011). In 1965 the Mongolian delegation to the World Health Organization made its own request to remove the terminology from all publications, which set a global precedent for ongoing national-level conversations (Howard-Jones 1979).

Not everyone I met in Jordan felt strongly about the unacceptability of *mongholi,* and few were familiar with the "commingling and interarticulation of 'race,' 'disability,' and 'chemistry'" that can be discerned through a critical reading of Down syndrome's history (Chen 2016, 236). My interlocutors described *mongholi* as a local insult with unclear racial connotations,[16] and they sought to situate Down syndrome in a medicalized and tentatively biosocial landscape of conditions connected to frameworks of disability or disease.[17] They contrasted Down syndrome with autism (*tawuhhud* or *idtirab tayf al-tawahhud*; autism spectrum disorder) in ways that revealed stereotypes associated with each, which they further distinguished from cerebral palsy (*shallal damaghi*), a condition with well-established local advocacy networks. I also encountered widespread references to *dumur al-ʿaql,* which translates to "cerebral atrophy," although people did not use more medicalized terms for brain (*damagh/ mukh*) in this context. *Mongholi* was not, however, the only contested term that I encountered during my fieldwork.

Abu Yousef, a university professor and the father of a toddler with Down syndrome, occasionally accompanied his wife and son to early intervention sessions at Al-Nur. I had previously met his wife on several occasions, so she introduced us and asked me to describe my project. Using a pitch that had not previously drawn scrutiny, I explained that my research examined the relationship between *iʿaqa ʿaqliyya* (intellectual disability) and culture. At the time, many people who employed disability language also used the phrase *i'aqa 'aqliyya* to describe Down syndrome.[18] Widely translated as "intellect" or "reason" (but also sometimes as "mental") 'aql serves as a "canonical concept . . . in Islamic philosophy, theology and jurisprudence" (Akrami 2017, 63). A "critical social sense" (Abu Lughod 1986, 124), 'aql grounds constructions of personhood in the philosophical, cultural, and material conditions that configure Jordanian bodyminds. Children, for example, do not possess full 'aql. Given the incompleteness of their 'aql, they should neither be held fully accountable for their actions nor taken too seriously when accounting for their wrongdoings.[19] In practice, people use 'aql to parse various distinctions: Human possess 'aql, while nonhuman animals do not; men are more reliable in using 'aql than women; elites demonstrate 'aql by behaving according to standards of decorum that non-elites lack (Hughes 2017; Meneley 1995; Peletz 1994).

When I shared this description of my research with Abu Yousef, he practically recoiled. "'I'aqa 'aqliyya?" His voice acquired a notably sharper edge. "Is that what we're calling Down syndrome now? Why not a learning or developmental delay" (ta'akhur ta'alimi aw namawi)? I immediately wondered whether I had committed a linguistic or cultural error. How had I managed to avoid doing so until that conversation? While Abu Yousef preferred the language of "delay," the term *i'aqa dhihniyya*, also translated as "intellectual" or "mental," has become the standard in Jordanian legal and advocacy settings. Jordan's previous disability rights law (No. 31 of 2007) defined a person with a disability as anyone with a partial or complete impairment, which could be *jasmiyya* (physical), *nafsiyya* (psychological), or *'aqliyya* (mental) in nature, but Law No. 20 of 2017 omits any reference to 'aql. Instead it defines disability in terms of physical (*jasadiyya*), sensory (*hassiya*), intellectual (*dhihniyya*), mental (*dhihniyya*), psychological (*nafsiyya*), or neurological (*'asabiyya*) impairment. The English translation differentiates between "intellectual" and "mental," while the Arabic version uses the dhihniyya for both.[20] The Arabic version of the CRPD distinguishes between 'aqliyya (translated as "mental") and dhihniyya (translated as "intellectual"), but other popular sources, including the U.N. page on World Down Syndrome Day, Al Jazeera, and the Facebook pages on Down syndrome advocacy initiatives based in Arabic-speaking countries, continue to use 'aqliyya. Charting changes around 'aql/iyya reveals reciprocities between language and disabled personhood, which is perhaps why my choice of words so deeply troubled Abu Yusuf.[21] Questioning Yusuf's 'aql could undermine his parents' efforts to maintain their son's access to a normative "masculine trajectory" (Ghannam 2013), a point I will return to in chapters 5 and 6.

Law. On the heels of the UN's Decade of Disabled Persons (1983–1992), Jordan passed Law No. 12 on the Welfare of Disabled Persons (1993). While grounded in a medical model of disability and lacking a rights-based approach, the law's mere existence and the legislative will behind it, set Jordan apart in the region. The country is home to several outstanding centers for special education and rehabilitation, although the best options are prohibitively expensive and concentrated in Amman. Most of these organizations operate through a model of segregated services, but they have spent decades raising awareness and facilitating community outreach under otherwise challenging conditions. Some, like the Al-Hussein Society–Jordan Center for Training and Inclusion, are actively involved in shifting disability paradigms. Established in 1971 and formerly known as the Al-Hussein Society for Rehabilitation, their recent name change signals their intentional realignment with current best principles.

Jordan embraced the CRPD as a blueprint for its own legislation. It was one of the first countries to sign the convention and its optional protocol, and it was the first Arab country to complete the ratification process. In the two decades since, it has executed two major legislative overhauls. First, it passed Law No. 31 of 2007 on the Rights of Persons with Disabilities (during the Arab Decade of Disabled Persons, 2003–2012). Ten years later that law was repealed and replaced by Law No. 20 of 2017 on the Rights of Persons with Disabilities. Law No. 20 is the region's first disability law grounded in the principle of antidiscrimination, and it strictly adheres to the social model in defining disability, rectifying a major weakness of its predecessor (Demeyere 2022).

Law No. 20 established the charter for the Higher Council for the Rights of Persons with Disabilities (HCD), which is responsible for managing implementation and compliance among all ministries that the provisions of Law No. 20 impact. The HCD's mandate is formidably vast. It oversees existing policies, proposes new laws and regulations, provides technical support to ministries, monitors and evaluates disability-related activities across the kingdom, and it is legally obligated to publish its activities in an annual report. Law No. 20 also assigned the HCD responsibility for developing a new system of disability identification cards, a process that requires obtaining medical reports from one of four official diagnosis centers run by the Ministry of Health.[22] During the COVID-19 pandemic, the HCD coordinated with government ministries on a number of pandemic-related matters, including vaccine access, distance-learning procedures, mental health awareness, and compliance with quarantine and lockdown procedures.

The HCD also hints at particularities of disability advocacy in Jordan. While financially and administratively independent, the council's president is appointed by a Royal Decree upon recommendation by the prime minister. Members of the board of trustees are also made by appointment, while the board's quota requirements ensure the representation of people with disabilities, family members of people with disabilities, and disability experts. The current president, Prince Mired bin Raed, also serves as chair for the National Committee for Demining and Rehabilitation and is a special envoy to the CRPD. His father,

Prince Ra'ed bin Zeid, served as president of the Higher Council for the Affairs of Persons with Disabilities, which was created under the auspices of Law No. 30 of 2007, until Prince Mired took over in 2014.[23] The Zeids boast impeccable educational degrees from top Western universities and matching career qualifications. Like other members of the extended Hashemite family, they serve as respected civic and humanitarian leaders. Yet they are usually installed in these roles by the king, and their pervasive influence demonstrates the monarchy's entrenchment in Jordan's distinctly nonoppositional civic sector.[24]

Since the early 2000s, the number of Civil Society Organizations (CSOs) registered in Jordan has more than tripled, growing from approximately 1,500 in 2008 to over 4,600 only eight years later (USAID 2016). CSOs function as critical service providers across the country, but their massive proliferation speaks more to the ongoing impacts of structural adjustment programs than the potential liberalization of Jordan's political system. The notable rise of family societies and associations, where kin groups organize and register themselves as NGOs, is worth noting (Baylouny 2008). As subsidies on basic goods and services are absorbed by a prohibitively expensive private sector or disappear entirely, family societies facilitate access to capital, work and travel opportunities, and other forms of emergency support. In doing so, they re-entrench (but also transform) kin-based relations of patronage and debt while reconfiguring public-private divides.[25]

Whether based on kinship or other identities and affiliations, CSOs in Jordan tend to couch their objectives in terms of charity, humanitarianism, and development.[26] The aversion to explicitly political or critical language is not unintentional. As a legal prerequisite to existence, CSOs are forbidden from engaging in "political activities"—a term that Law No. 51 on Societies of 2008 (and its 2009 amendments) fails to define. This vagueness reinforces the registry board's authority to dissolve societies or to deny initial applications without justification, while operating a CSO without approval from the board amounts to a criminal offense (ICNL 2024). Both Law No. 51 and its amendments limit the ability of societies to receive foreign funding, a measure justified as necessary to counterterrorism efforts.[27] These sociopolitical conditions complicate Global North–driven theorizing about disability models and politics, and they influence how organizations position themselves on the ground and in relation to the communities that they both belong to and serve.

Despite developing and passing progressive laws, the government has struggled to actualize its own policies. A blistering 2019 communiqué issued by Human Rights Watch noted that several key ministries charged with implementing Law No. 20—which included those of the Interior, Municipal Affairs, Tourism and Antiquities, Transport, Digital Economy and Entrepreneurship, and Awqaf and Islamic Affairs—allocated no money to disability provisions in 2018 or 2019. The Ministry of Education's Strategic Plan for 2018–2022 outlined one disability-related objective—increasing the enrollment of students with disabilities (further broken down into four key subcomponents)—but allocated no portion of its budget to this goal. Instead, it dedicated 0.4 percent to "special education services." In the words of the Human Rights Watch deputy director for the Middle East and North Africa region, "Jordan's disability rights law is great on paper, but it means nothing for people with disabilities if the government will not put it into practice" (Human Rights Watch 2019). This gap between "ink on paper" and reality became especially clear in the context of education.

INCLUSION: LIVING INK ON PAPER

In spring 2014 I attended several events held to mark World Down Syndrome Day, which happens every year on March 21 (a date chosen by Down syndrome advocacy organizations to highlight and celebrate three copies of chromosome 21).[28] The program featured recreational and educational activities for children and families, and the latter included presentations about recent developments in disability rights and law. Families attended these events with different motivations. Some welcomed a reason to get their kids out of the house and into a welcoming space where they could play with their peers, hopefully under the watchful eyes of volunteer chaperones. Others sought opportunities to gain a better handle on changing laws and policies and to learn from fellow parents and invited speakers. They also became venues for airing shared grievances.

Toward the end of a talk by a renowned expert on inclusive education, the conversation between two audience members rose to what sounded like an argument, and their raised voices drew the attention of those within earshot. One of the participants in this exchange, a middle-aged man, grew so frustrated that he jumped up from his seat and made a dramatic exit from the auditorium, yelling loudly. I turned to the other participant, whom I knew from the Al-Nur Society, and asked what happened. The man with whom she had been chatting was the father of a boy with Down syndrome, and he had grown increasingly infuriated by the gap between the speakers' claims and reality (*al-ard al-waqiʿ*). He could not afford to pay private school fees, so he deemed all this talk about inclusion useless. This was because, as my companion explained, "private school is the only way to access any sort of inclusive program."

Article 24 of the CRPD states that "parties shall ensure an inclusive education system at all levels" (2006a). Jordan's Articles 17–23 of Law No. 20 of 2017 address different facets of this directive, beginning with the declaration that "it is forbidden to exclude someone from any educational institution on the basis of, or because of, disability." Yet during the 2018–2019 academic year, disabled students represented 1.9 percent of the 1.4 million children enrolled in school at the primary level across Jordan, and 79 percent of school-aged disabled children had no access to education of any kind (Humanity and Inclusion 2022). During conferences and in professional settings, I witnessed audience members express visible shock when receiving these and other disability-related education statistics, as they dramatically countered Jordan's reputation for educational excellence.[29] Inclusion and education were so closely linked that whenever I mentioned "inclusion" (*damaj*), people automatically assumed I was referring to education rather than the term's broader connotations or possibilities.

Within educational contexts, however, inclusion provoked considerable debate. Few families questioned the importance of educating children with disabilities, but some argued that the discourse of "inclusion" failed to mitigate how class and capital mediate children's access to education of different qualities and kinds. Among "first-generation" champions of inclusive education (Scandinavia, the United States, Canada, England), family advocacy groups were key drivers of policy change (Artiles et al. 2011). "Second-generation" countries, however, which include the majority of the ninety-two signatories to the 1994 Salamanca Statement (and Framework for Action on Special Needs Education), have relied on top-down initiatives. The resultant shortcomings manifest in widespread discrepancies between policy and practice (Artiles et al. 2011; Singal and Muthukrishna 2014), which become glaringly obvious in the case of Jordan (Benson 2020). Private schools have historically proven more willing to experiment with inclusion, for a price, but even families with ample financial resources have questioned the associated costs.

The topic of inclusive education provoked considerable ambivalence for Umm Reham. An affluent stay-at-home mother to three children, Umm Reham wanted the best for her daughter (Reham). Yet in hindsight she wondered whether it offered them the "best" outcomes. She equivocated on the question value, explaining: "You feel in the schools, the time she spends in the class with the rest of the normal girls [*al-binat normal*]; it's useless. I feel that they are on one side, and Reham is on her side. . . . The schools Reham went to take the fees for her class plus 50 percent extra because of the help. So, we were paying around 2,000 dinar per year. It was better, but she also wasn't benefiting when she was in the [integrated] class. . . . I mean, she doesn't have friends. You feel that most people who know her, they feel sorry for her, not taking her as a friend. They pity her but they don't really like her."

Subverting the normative association of inclusion with a progressive and rights-based stance, Umm Reham wondered if the laborious and expensive pursuit of inclusive education—40 percent of Jordanian households' yearly expenditures fell between 5,000 and 10,000 dinar in 2018—actually reflected her own struggle to truly accept Reham's Down syndrome.[30] By avoiding special education centers, had she denied Reham the opportunity to develop meaningful friendships with peers with Down syndrome? "Maybe I don't want her to have Down syndrome friends," she mused aloud. "I don't know. I don't know." The thread of acceptance runs through this ethnography, and Umm Reham's use of the term highlights the plurality of its possible referents. She questioned whether her resistance to disability-centered spaces (which, for people with intellectual disabilities like Down syndrome, primarily took the form of special education centers) further isolated Reham over time, especially as her classmates moved on to college, work, and marriage.

Jordan's disability imaginaries, as reflected through law and policy, diminish the material and technological dimensions of accessibility that pose serious obstacles for students with disabilities. After the Syrian popular revolution against Bashar al-Assad (2011–2012) spiraled into a devastating civil war (2012–2024), a significant number of Jordanian public schools began running double shifts for refugee children, an immense undertaking that intensified strains on the educational system and further complicated the issue of reform. Rectifying the barriers that disabled students face requires direct financial investment, while the cultural and pedagogical shifts required for truly inclusive education demand broad transformations in teacher training and curriculum development (and more financial investment).[31] As "ink on paper," inclusion reveals gaps between conventions and laws, on the one hand, and the inequalities and infrastructural breakdowns that shape actual schools on the other.

The Ministry of Education's 2018–2022 Strategic Plan demonstrates how culturalism shapes extant disability imaginaries. The report explains a notable gender gap in the already low rates of intellectually disabled students enrolled in school as a result of families' attempts to keep disabled girls at home for "cultural reasons" (Ministry of Education 2018, 9 [24 in Ar. version]).[32] This mirrors a fact sheet produced by Humanity and Inclusion (Handicap International) that cites "prevailing negative attitudes of families and communities towards disability" as a major obstacle to educational access, attitudes they describe as intensifying among Jordanian families in poverty and Syrian refugees (2022). Yet the very same sheet quotes a mother expressing hope that her son will one day have access to schooling and a Syrian father explaining that he tried to enroll his son, but the principal rejected him. The qualitative data informing these official representations contradicts the assertion that "culture" is primarily responsible for families choosing to "keep" disabled children at home and out of school.

Exclusionary realities of capitalism, which configure education as a commodity for purchase rather than a right available to all, intensified doubts about inclusion. During the question-and-answer session at the World Down Syndrome Day talk where the disgruntled father fled the auditorium, many frustrated parents chose to stay and air their complaints. An older woman, flanked by her husband and their adult daughter with Down syndrome, made her way to the microphone and stated that no matter what the law might claim or strive to achieve, only private schools accepted disabled children. As she spoke I noticed a man sitting in front of me nod his head in a vigorous show of support while rubbing his fingers together to make the sign for cash. Eventually, the "dialogue session" took a turn; agitated parents got to their feet and began yelling at the guest speaker, who remained stranded onstage: "Where? Where can we put our children?!" they shouted. "Tell us which school will take them, and we're there."

Amid this collective outburst, a mother I knew from the Al-Nur Society, Umm Abdullah, stood up and announced to the crowd, "Give me a classroom, and I will teach them!" A round of applause followed her invitation. Later, Umm Abdullah explained that despite her commitment, she did not see inclusion as a straightforward process. She told me: "Look, at first I wanted inclusion. I want my son to be included. But there need to be specific preparations for it to hap-pen. There must be early intervention, and at five or six years old there should be a class for . . . for . . . Down. They have Down syndrome. *Khalas*! Accept that they have Down syndrome [Kuni mutaqabbaleh humeh Down]! Afterwards, I would integrate him, even if it meant him entering school a year or two late. The important thing is that my son has to be ready to handle it." When parents like Umm Abdullah questioned whether inclusion should happen automatically or could unfold similarly for every child, their caution risked becoming evidence of cultural "backwardness." Not pursuing inclusive educational programming, advocates argued, was tantamount to "hiding" a child at home or in a segregated center. Parents who disagreed, or who expressed hesitation like Um Abdullah, often identified as fierce defenders of their child's right to education, to friend-ship, and to developing fulfilling lives. They differentiated, however, between education and schooling. Valuing the former without qualification, they main-tained serious doubts about the latter. They did not hesitate to denounce structural barriers to education, lament the lack of quality schools, or express dismay at the disproportionately high illiteracy rates among disabled children and adults, but they remained unconvinced that inclusion offered the best solution.[33]

The (neo)liberal operationalization of education as a tool for individual eco-nomic betterment and national development rests on the assumption that education will lead to higher rates of participation in the workforce. This under-standing of educational reform as critical for the kingdom's economic (and thus political) stability is reflected in how Jordan's National Human Resource Devel-opment (HRD) Strategy for 2016–2025 anchored the Ministry of Education's 2018–2022 Strategic Plan. Developed by an expert committee at the king's behest, the HRD is a product of Jordan's Education Reform for Knowledge Economy Project, a multidonor initiative created to realize the 2002 Vision Forum for the Future of Education in Jordan (Ministry of Education 2013). Many Jordanians agree with this premises. Whether alongside or in lieu of more abstract ideals, they value education as a pathway toward upward economic mobility, or at least as a preventive against downward mobility.[34]

Umm Reham connected her misgivings about inclusive education to the inevi-table passage of time and her family's interwoven life transitions, anticipating this progression through economic calculations and classed assumptions about purpose. Without hesitation, she positioned her sons as moving along a straightforward path: They would go to college, establish their careers, and get married and start families. Reham's path, however, remained less certain. "I always tell my husband, why don't you start a business so Reham and I can work there? Even a supermarket! Let's do something. I don't know if people employ them [people with disabilities], but I think we're probably the best option to find her a job." Like so many parents, Umm Reham wondered what kind of education could provide Reham with a reliable cash flow or, at the very least, with goals and a structure for her everyday routine. Unlike the many girls and young women who embedded their educational trajectories in marital and maternal aspirations, or vice versa (Adely 2012a), Umm Reham assumed that Reham would never become a wife or mother. This assumption drove her to focus on work as a meaningful pursuit, a point I will return to in chapter 6.

"ISN'T THIS INCLUSION [TOO]?"

A conversation between Kawthar, a special educator, and Umm Zayd, the mother of a toddler with Down syndrome, revealed some of the "friction" generated through encounters with inclusion (Tsing 2005). Several families that I knew from Al-Nur had gathered to attend a launch party for a new cultural center that boasted a coveted playground designed with accessibility in mind and a semigreen space. While chatting and enjoying the snacks, Kawthar asked Umm Zayd if she planned to find an inclusive program for Zayd once he reached kindergarten age. Umm Zayd expressed considerable anxiety about whether she could find a school that would meet her standards. Kawthar nodded sympathetically. To demonstrate why she did not think Umm Zayd's hesitation was inherently problematic, she asked the following questions:

KAWTHAR: Do you hide Zayd from your family?
UMM ZAYD: No, of course not!
KAWTHAR: Everyone knows [that he has Down syndrome]?
UMM ZAYD: Everyone knows.
KAWTHAR: Do you take him places with you or leave him at home [*fil bayt*]?
UMM ZAYD: We take him everywhere.
KAWTHAR: Isn't this inclusion? Why do we have to have educational inclusion? Why is that the standard for what inclusion means?

Kawthar's provocations did not hinge solely on her doubts about the feasibility of actualizing inclusion. Instead, they articulated deeper concerns about the purpose and value of education in today's world. Parents of the children with whom she worked shared many of these concerns, especially as the shifting hierarchies of knowledge and skill valued by today's labor markets create new barriers for potential workers with intellectual disabilities. So, too, did the bitter truth that even the best education could fail to guarantee a reasonable salary or any employment at all.

Grounded in the core axes of Jordan's broader disability imaginaries—hiding and inclusion—Kawthar and Umm Zayd oriented themselves toward alternative spaces and outcomes. They prioritized securing their children's belonging to kinship futures rather than the country's increasingly strained education system and worsening labor market. In these efforts, "the bayt [was] fundamental." This is what Umm Iyad, the mother of a four-year-old with Down syndrome, affirmed to a group of women who had gathered one morning in the reception room of the Al-Nur Society for an open discussion. "Without the family," she continued, "individual rights will not be realized." *Al-bayt* can refer to the physical domestic structure of a housing unit and smaller neo- or patrilocal settlements, but it also encompasses the emotional and symbolic resonances of home and family (Hughes 2021; Meneley 1996). Fewer Jordanians today live in extended patrilocal arrangements, but al-bayt also covers the nuclear family unit and extends to broader political groupings like the Hashemites, who rule as a family and interpolate their subjects through what some have described as "house politics" (Shryock and Howell 2001).

While attending a support group hosted by an organization in one of Amman's poorest, most vulnerable eastern neighborhoods, I listened to a different group of mothers discuss change in the context of disability rights. An older woman, pondering the question of how to transform society, volunteered the following directive and strongly echoed Umm Iyad: "First yourself, then the bayt, then the neighbors, then the society." Her words brought me back to my early conversation with Abu Yehya and the map he drew around the "the most important thing," acceptance: "The mother, the father, the family, neighbors, society." Across class and geographic divides, many families oriented themselves toward more sociocentric and domestically driven understandings of which spaces mattered and how social change progressed. In no way obviating the importance of "the individual," they coordinated this unit relative to the primacy of the bayt, before connecting outward (to neighbors, society, and its institutions).

EXPANSIVE IMAGINARIES

The disability imaginaries I outline in this chapter framed how my interlocutors made sense of me and my research, even as I tried to resist their culturalist underpinnings. Because I am neither myself disabled nor caring for a disabled family member and given that I lacked professional training in special education or rehabilitative sciences, some people found my interest in disability quite perplexing.

Consequently, I found myself being made intelligible as supposed evidence of the high standard of care that people imagined to be seamlessly accessible in "the West." Disability rights and awareness must be well rooted in the United States, according to this logic, if I traveled all the way to Jordan to embark on such a project.

In this way I became another diagnostic marker of local cultural flaws, and some parents or teachers used their encounters with me to lament what they saw as a lack of volunteerism or sense of civic responsibility in Jordan. For my part, I tried to convey how radically unequal state-level commitments and implementation strategies made it impossible to describe a cohesive picture of disability rights or accessibility in the United States. But unless my audience was familiar with these disparities firsthand, they remained skeptical of my counterarguments. At the same time, this imagined world of better support and services presented a peculiar paradox. Put simply, many of my interlocutors expressed polite bewilderment at why a country so seemingly indifferent to the sanctity of human life—as evidenced by the death, destruction, and disablement it has forged across the region—valued the dignity of its citizens with disabilities.

While navigating these imaginaries, I frequently found myself on the receiving end of questions about U.S. disability rights legislation, accumulating a running list of research topics about the Americans with Disabilities Act and the Individuals with Disabilities Education Act. My fieldwork upended my own assumptions about Down syndrome and forced me to acknowledge how ableist concepts of intelligence and capacity lingered in my constructions of personhood. My relatively prior isolation from people with intellectual disabilities, especially given the extensive amount of time I have spent in private institutions of secondary and higher education (Dolmage 2017; Price 2011), became painfully apparent through this process. It also heightened my appreciation for the state-market interactions that shape accessible and inclusive schools and workplaces.

Ultimately, Jordan's disability imaginaries revolved around promises of material, social, and moral development—however incompletely realized. These progress-driven narratives offered a sharp contrast to the abundance of local and regional narratives that center on deterioration, stagnation, and hopelessness. Yet "progress" was not innocent, as evidenced by colonialist and culturalist logics of comparison that far too easily diminished the complexities of Jordan's emerging disability worlds. Dominant disability imaginaries, moreover, led to neither homogeneity nor consensus. Instead, they fueled diverse and conflicting expressions of hope and critique, which surfaced repeatedly throughout the making of Down syndrome I explore in the chapters to come.

3 · AFTERSHOCKS

"Mothers don't cause Down syndrome!"

Umm Zayna and I chatted quietly, waiting for the setting sun and the call to prayer signal that the iftar, or the evening meal that breaks each day's fast during the month of Ramadan, could commence. Appearing somewhat lost in thought, she cast her eyes around the room and studied the scene. Hosted by the Al-Nur Society, the event brought together mothers and children with Down syndrome, as well as fathers, siblings, volunteers, and friends hailing from all corners of Amman's vast sprawl and even some neighboring governorates. The tightly packed reception room buzzed with the anticipation that peaks just before sundown after a day of fasting, a practice undertaken by those old enough and well enough to participate.

Many of the women present knew each other well, having spent years or even decades seeking services for their children; they were acquaintances, allies, and sometimes friends. Those journeying from east to west during the city's most infamous traffic season had to plan their routes and departures wisely. Attending this kind of iftar also meant accepting a boxed to-go meal, which typically failed to compete with the family favorites that women prepared in their own kitchens and by their own hands (or, at the very least, managed and delegated under their own watchful eyes). Nevertheless, and despite the disincentives, many chose to make the trip. They were motivated in large part by children who, just like their mothers, developed meaningful relationships through the Down syndrome social networks expanding across Jordan's capital.

"I suppose," Umm Zayna began, thinking aloud more than speaking to anyone in particular, "that I'm the oldest mother here . . ." Her voice trailed off. She refocused her gaze on her baby daughter, Zayna, who was fast asleep in the crook of one arm, while absentmindedly adjusting the folds of a flower-patterned hijab with her free hand. Umm Zayna did not need to finish this thought, however, before she was met by a chorus of "tsks" and impatient vocalizations. Umm Munir, the mother of a toddler with Down syndrome and a longer-term participant at Al-Nur, threw her arms toward Umm Zayna, the long sleeves of her jilbab shaking as she gestured emphatically. "Ya ukhti, the mother does not cause

Down syndrome" (Ya ukhti, al-umm ma tasabbab Down)![1] Umm Munir placed extra emphasis on "does not cause" for dramatic emphasis, while several women seated within earshot nodded vigorously in agreement.

Umm Zayna's concern about being the oldest woman in the room suggested her familiarity—and her concern for others' familiarity—with the most significant medical risk factor for Down syndrome: advanced maternal age (AMA); this risk factor persists despite the fact that the majority of babies with Down syndrome are born to women under thirty-five (the threshold for AMA).[2] The exchange between Umm Zayna and Umm Munir also gestured to a broader perception—whether spoken or left implicit—that even beyond medical factors, *women* somehow bore unique responsibility for their child's disability. It was this heaviness that prompted Umm Munir to urgently rebut Umm Zayna's unfinished thought. On a deeper level, questions about *why* Down syndrome occurred and *what* might be "responsible" blurred into questions of *who* could or should be held accountable. They reflected how people related to Down syndrome as not only nonordinary but abnormal, as something that demanded further scrutiny.

In this chapter I focus on the postdiagnosis moment and the emotions that surfaced as mothers—and sometimes fathers—shared memories from this stage of life. The intensity of these conversations sometimes took parents by surprise. If a voice began to tremble or eyes suddenly shone brightly with tears, I always offered to change directions or stop the conversation entirely. My interlocutors ignored these invitations, using humor to recalibrate and regain control of their narrative. But tentative pauses, heavy sighs, and words that got caught in the back of the throat helped me appreciate how forcefully shock reverberated through relations, even when it eventually dissipated into the more mundane rhythms of everyday life.[3]

IN AND AFTER SHOCK

Umm Zayna had only begun building the kinds of relationships that convinced Umm Munir to brave Amman's formidable traffic and forgo a homecooked meal that warm summer evening. She was immersed in a period of life that my interlocutors considered the most difficult, when the unknowns of a newly received diagnosis outweighed the Down syndrome wisdom gained through lived experience and time. Whether the mother of a newborn or a child fully grown, most women described those earliest months and years after their child's diagnosis as a period of *sadma*, or shock.

The birth of a baby invited parents and kin to imagine and dream about the future, but the birth of a baby with Down syndrome generated intensely future-oriented questions. What would happen between spouses? What would happen to the marriage prospects of siblings and cousins? What would happen to that baby, once grown, after their siblings and cousins married? Would they marry? Would they work? Where would they live? How would they be kept safe after their parents passed? Who was most likely to die first? Families wondered about the person their child would become, and they wondered about the kind of family they would become. They imagined these possible futures—kinship futures—through the presence and absence of lineal and affinal relationships. In working through the throes of shock, the weight of kin relations came into sharper relief than the specificities of Down syndrome or the singular individual living "under its description" (Martin 2007, xviii).

The anxiety that women experienced while anticipating the reactions of husbands, extended family members, neighbors, and even strangers attested to the stakes of giving birth to a child with visible, marked forms of difference. Few of the women I knew well ultimately experienced life-altering conflict or ostracism because of their child's Down syndrome, at least not to the degree they initially feared. Some pursued unexpected educational opportunities. Others took up new roles as advocates and organizers. All experienced the joys and grief that accompany parenthood in its many stages. But shock linked the more distant memories of mothers with grown children to the more proximate experiences of mothers with young children. Whether from firsthand knowledge or via second-hand stories, shock revealed a vexing contradiction: the capacity of close relations to inflict the deepest cuts of estrangement. What did it mean that kin could not be counted on to accept disability among their own? While families criticized and positioned themselves against the anxieties that permeated diagnostic after-shocks, they did not dismiss them. They saw these fears as an understandable (but misguided) outcome of how ties between kin—as reproduced and cemented through bonds of marriage—are critical to survival and well-being. In their respective roles as spouses, women and men had unequal resources available to mitigate shock, which potentially put them in conflict. In some cases it led to marital breakdown. But as an allied unit, spouses could—and many did—work together to manage their broader kin and social networks.[4]

Shock appeared nearly ubiquitously across my interlocutors' narratives, but I use "diagnosis" as a shorthand for the variety of paths that parents traversed to recognize and confirm their child's Down syndrome. Official diagnosis involved a formal confirmation of chromosomal difference, but the journey might begin with an offhand comment from a friend, a Facebook search, or even by consulting a biology textbook.[5] Diagnosis generated a broad scope of labels and predictions, which ranged from delicate discussions of developmental delay to brazen pronouncements of intellectual impairment or "slowness."[6] Some women received more dire prognostications, with medical staff or family members preparing them to witness profound impairment and early death.[7] Others received few concrete details or no mention of Down syndrome at all. While the negative extremes left much to be desired, even women who received compassionate treatment, accurate information, and unconditional family support conveyed the intensity of shock through their bodies and words.

Diagnosis, across its variable formations, did not define subsequent possibilities of making Down syndrome. In the worst-case scenario, Down syndrome could precipitate a potential crisis of kinship for reasons I explore in the sections to come. But women also marshaled their power as wives and mothers (and as sisters, grandmothers, and cousins, and as professionals and experts) to advocate for themselves and their children. This entailed challenging an extant logic that positioned Down syndrome as a collective risk or hazard. To do so they harnessed overlapping moral rubrics (Deeb and Harb 2013; Hamdy 2012) of kinship, biomedicine, and Islam, but Down syndrome also prompted them to critically reassess the authority of their rubrics. Primarily considered interpretive instruments, rubrics bring ways of seeing, being, and *making* into the world. They positioned diagnosis as an open-ended catalyst for making Down syndrome through everyday practices of care.

DIAGNOSTIC TEMPORALITIES

In reflecting on the journey to and from diagnosis, women mobilized shock as a noun (I was in a state of shock), an active verb (it shocked me), and a reflexive verb (I was shocked). For some, the postnatal character of diagnosis amplified its intensity. For others, the paradoxical combination of authority and uncertainty carried by any diagnosis made shock inevitable, irrespective of the mode or timing of delivery. After all, what could a label attached to an infant really convey about a person-to-be or about lives to come? Given these contradictions, the relative merits of prenatal diagnostic technologies, which are available but unevenly implemented across Jordan's well-developed health care system, generated considerable disagreement.

Because trisomy in chromosome 21 is detectable through screening and diagnostic technologies, Down syndrome communities have long existed in the crosshairs between movements for reproductive and disability rights, with the latter at risk of becoming weaponized in efforts to restrict the former. Yet far less attention has been paid to how communities navigate these intersections outside Western European and North American contexts. None of the women I met received a prenatal diagnosis of Down syndrome. None had received any kind of prenatal indicator or confirmation of fetal difference despite the availability and relative accessibility of prenatal health care across the country.[8] In the reception room at Al-Nur, during the public lectures and celebrations that I attended across the capital, and in my more formal interviews, prenatal diagnostics emerged as a subjunctive presence (Sargent 2020). Sometimes raised explicitly and other times left implicit, a hypothetical question haunted these discussions.

"What would I have done," women wondered to themselves, to each other, and to me, "if I had known?"

In Jordan, pregnancy is thoroughly medicalized but unevenly biomedicalized (Clarke et al. 2003) because of inconsistencies in the availability and implementation of new medical technologies.[9] Cost can pose a significant hurdle, as private insurance companies do not always cover a second trimester ultrasound (Thekrallah et al. 2013, 76).[10] For women using public insurance, the limited availability of equipment and high demand for services present similar obstacles (Thekrallah et al. 2013, 76). Discrepancies between the procedures and tests available in private practices versus public and nongovernmental organization–based clinics have also been reported (Maffi 2013). Even when prenatal diagnostic tests are ostensibly available, doctors may nevertheless avoid promoting them.[11] Yet precisely because most women routinely encountered biomedical institutions and actors during pregnancy, they expressed surprise that doctors did not "catch" their child's Down syndrome beforehand. Some specifically mentioned completing ultrasounds or lab work as part of their antenatal care routine, while others made vague references to medical experts without specifying tests or technologies.[12]

The existence of prenatal diagnostic technologies produces increasingly inescapable subjunctive conditions, but legal structures and moral norms shape the realities that these technologies can conjure. Jordan's penal code prohibits abortion, while Article 12 of the Public Health Act (Law No. 47) of 2008 and Article 21 of the Medical Constitution recognize "danger to the mother's health" as legitimate grounds for termination (Ministry of Health 2008; Nimri 2016, 2019). Contradictory interpretations and variable public perceptions of the law's legitimacy, however, contribute to ongoing debates about the legality of pregnancy termination and which extenuating circumstances prove valid. The field of Islamic bioethics generates an even wider range of stances on the permissibility of abortion than the national laws operating in Jordan and across the Southwest Asia and North Africa (SWANA) region.[13]

Fatwas, or legally nonbinding edicts issued by religious scholars, carry notable moral authority, and they are meant to guide and inform the spirit of Jordanian law. As early as 1993, Jordan's Council of Iftaa' ruled it permissible to terminate a fetus prior to four months of gestation, with both parents' consent, if doctors determined that it suffered from an impairment that would "make its life unstable" (Dar Al-Ifta' 2015). Medicalization of the fetus—and of disability by extension—has played a role in expanding access to abortion across the region, with Iran, Kuwait, Qatar, Saudi Arabia, Tunisia, and the United Arab Emirates all recognizing termination based on fetal impairment as religiously and legally permissible (Maffi and Tonnessen 2019; Newman 2018).[14] Fatwas inform legal philosophy and everyday moral deliberations, but they are not synonymous with law, and their subtleties do not always permeate popular discourse. Nor does ostensible legality equate to practical accessibility (Dabash and Roudi-Fahimi 2008).[15] Shifting hospital policies and spousal consent laws configure abortion as a collective decision that belongs to medical practitioners, husbands, and extended family members rather than an autonomous pregnant person.

The ethical and legal complexities of assisted reproductive technologies offer compelling lessons in the construction of kinship (Clarke 2009; Inhorn 2012, 2015; Inhorn and Tremayne 2016), but they also create capacity for kinship's denial (Wahlberg and Gammeltoft 2018). Some women asserted that it was better not to know and that one *should not* know. This technological refusal placed kinship and disability beyond the subjunctive "what-ifs" summoned by prenatal diagnostics. Others, however, disagreed. While worried about making the "right" choice, they advocated for having a choice to make. Across this divide, women viewed prenatal diagnosis as a source of suffering, either by enabling access to knowledge about something potentially unchangeable or by enabling intervention into something better left unknowable. In the context of my research, however, the postnatal timing of diagnosis shaped how families managed shock and subsequently worked to make Down syndrome in the earliest months and years of their child's life.

HERITABILITY

The urgency with which Umm Zayna and Umm Munir treated the question of Down syndrome's etiology reflected broader concerns about the connections that make and distinguish kin from nonkin and how affinal ties differ from those forged through descent. Etiology often turned into discussions about *wuratha*, a term that stretches across meanings of heredity, legacy, inheritance, and transmission. The compound of *'ilm al-wuratha* (the science of wuratha), for example, is used to describe the contemporary field of genetics. I render wuratha here as *heritability*, both to set it apart from an extensive literature on Islamic inheritance law and to recognize its capacity to blur the boundaries between different kinds of bonds. In other words, the gloss of heritability acknowledges the expansive affordances of "inheritance" that coexisted and contradicted each other as people parsed matters and matter-ings of relatedness through Down syndrome (Carsten 2000).

In Jordan, heritability served as a potential indictment of family lineage, which made it a powerful moral rubric. In examining the ethics of organ donation in contemporary Egypt, the anthropologist Sherine Hamdy uses the concept of "political etiologies" to describe how people "make meaning out of illness and explain kidney disease in terms of the social, economic, and political ills afflicting Egypt as a whole" (2008, 554). The meanings that people in Jordan made out of Down syndrome lacked the state-centered focus of Hamdy's interlocutors and pivoted instead on heritability's more intimate and enduring "everyday biopolitics" (Fullwiley 2004). The moral rubric of heritability also surfaces prior to marriage when women relatives conduct their own diagnostic probing during the matchmaking process, asking pointed questions about the individual and familial health histories of prospective partners (Hughes 2015). An increasing focus on consanguineous marriage as a public health risk adds another layer to these everyday biopolitics, the ramifications of which I return to later in this chapter.[16]

When grappling with the stakes of heritability, patriarchal solidarities reinforced patrilineal ties. While both men and women participate in and experience the burdens of these systems, the latter remain more vulnerable. Women bear greater responsibility in representing and maintaining family reputation through their conduct, and the standards of appropriateness and respectability by which they are judged hinge on expectations around sexuality and sexual propriety, as well as other class-inflected ideals of femininity (Adely 2012a, 2012b, 2016; MacDougall 2021; Mahadeen 2013; Tobin 2016; Yessayan 2015). Women are responsible for continuing their husband's patriline—by bearing children—but they do not join this lineage. This can make them especially vulnerable to criticism and accusations of wrongdoing by husbands and in-laws, particularly in matters of reproduction and infertility (Inhorn 1994).[17]

My interlocutor Serene, a well-established special educator, advocate, and proud relative to a family member with Down syndrome, clarified this point for me. I had asked her about wuratha and whether she thought education on Down syndrome's genetics would diminish the stigma surrounding it. Contemplating the question, Serene responded with a mix of sarcasm and exasperation, but the lightness of her words did not mask the weight of her answer. "Arabs blame the mother when a daughter is born. We all know who is responsible for that second X chromosome! And still, they blame her!" Son preference, while by no means universal or without its vocal critics, likewise reveals mutual reinforcements between patriarchy and patrilineality. Even though the male's genetic contribution "determines" fetal sex, women may get "blamed" when a daughter is born or, more accurately, when they bear no sons. (Most women possess XX sex chromosomes, meaning they have only an X chromosome to give the fetus; the second X or Y is thus "determined" by the male contributor.)

Serene did not interpret gendered blame as a symptom of unfamiliarity with or an inability to comprehend a biogenetic account of fertilization. Instead, she highlighted a disconnect; biogenetic models, whether of fertilization or inheritance, coexist with other models. These circulate and comingle together through preexisting systems of power and inequality, which converge to position women as culpable for unexpected (and undesired) birth outcomes. In general, biogenetic explanations for chromosomal disorders appear to make a good deal of sense in Jordan, partly because chromosomal transmission follows pathways that overlap with the genealogical formulas that families use across the SWANA region to trace their histories and boundaries (Inhorn 2003; see also Clarke 2007; Samin 2015). Yet despite their relatively smooth uptake, important differences persist.

Biogenetics relies on notions of randomness and risk to convey why and how Down syndrome occurs. These concepts failed to defuse enduring concerns about heritable transmission or potential contagion. My interlocutor Hana elaborated further on how scientific ambiguity and patriarchy colluded through heritability. Hana was extremely close with her youngest brother, Jamal, over time growing into a role she described as akin to his second mother. They attended social events together, and she contributed to managing the logistics of his daily routine as much as her own career and family life allowed. In trying to convey the force and temporal reach of wuratha, Hana offered the following explanation: "There's this idea that when people marry their children in the future, if people come for their daughter, especially the daughter, maybe people will say, 'Ah her brother has Down syndrome . . . no no no. Maybe in the future she will also have a child with Down syndrome.' They think there's wuratha."

To convey the pervasiveness of this concern, she told me about a television program in which the hosts had stopped people on the streets of Amman to ask if they would marry a girl whose brother had Down syndrome. "Most people said no!" Hana exclaimed. "[The hosts] told them it's not inherited, and people said, 'Maybe it's inherited. Maybe not.' And some people said, 'Stay away. Why bring problems?'" Hana was perplexed and irritated by the interviewees' equivocation. For her, the answer was clear: Down syndrome is a chromosomal disorder, but it is not passed from parent to child. Given its nonheritability, why should having a relative with Down syndrome impinge on assessments of marriageability? For those interviewed during the television segment, the question clearly mattered, but the answer remained unclear. Slippage between inheritance, heredity, and heritability left respondents wary, so an ambiguous "maybe" persisted.

While biomedicine's individualizing capacities typically draw the ire of medical anthropologists, here they offered an authoritative narrative for casting doubt on Down syndrome's presumed heritability. By redrawing and contracting the body's boundaries, biomedicine could potentially contain problematic connections between kin. But it was an unpredictable and partial ally at best. The threat of transmissibility did not necessarily reflect a misunderstanding of genetics but attested to how moral dimensions of sickness and the contagiousness of kinship create precarious conditions for bodyminds deemed not healthy or not normal.[18] Even when people accepted that Down syndrome did not result from parent-child genetic transmission, other substances, qualities, and dangers (chromosomal or otherwise) could still pass through family lines. So etiological ambiguity introduced profound shocks into a social landscape where ties between lineal kin and those forged through marriage played critical roles in building one's sense of self, relations with others, and imagined futures. Given these limitations, families also drew on nonmedical sources of moral authority to reformat the rubric of heritability. Medical and genetic knowledge surfaced but never alone sufficed for absorbing the aftershocks of diagnosis and creating the foundations for life after shock.

DIAGNOSTIC FAULT LINES

I first met Umm Reham and her daughter Reham at a free medical event geared toward younger children and their families. Already in her late teens, Reham attracted intense interest from many of the parents in attendance. As she made her way around the room, offering greetings and inquiring about people's health, the open stares she received from some of the parents in the room started to make me uncomfortable. Reham, however, seemed unfazed. Watching other parents watch her so intently, I sensed that they saw Reham as a window into their own children's futures, and they closely studied her movements, speech, mannerisms, and manners.

While Reham jumped keenly into the setting, her mother held back. Taking note of the younger children in attendance, she began to realize that they had perhaps misread the intended audience for the event, but they stayed anyway. As Reham became more involved in programming at Al-Nur, I increasingly crossed paths with her and her mother. Eventually, I interviewed Umm Reham at an upscale mall in their neighborhood, and I later visited them at their family home. Recalling her initial days as a new mother nearly twenty years prior, Umm Reham reflected on her limited exposure to Down syndrome. "I saw people like her when I was younger," she recalled, switching between Arabic and English with an ease that indexed her class and educational status. "But I didn't know anything scientific about them, that their name was Down syndrome. I knew them like everyone knows them, as *mongholi*."

Umm Reham did not learn about Reham's Down syndrome prenatally or during the immediate postnatal period, but she remembered lingering on the shape of her newborn daughter's eyes. A month would pass, however, before her husband explained that Reham was born with an extra chromosome. Reham's doctor had in fact ordered diagnostic tests for her shortly after Reham was born, but he did not communicate his suspicions to both parents. Instead, he confirmed Reham's Down syndrome with her father (a point I return to below), who immediately called his mother-in-law for advice. Umm Reham's mother recommended they schedule a meeting to see the doctor as a family so the latter could explain the situation to Umm Reham. Until then, she advised her son-in-law to say nothing. Before he could organize the follow-up appointment, Umm Reham felt increasingly unsettled by what she described as "just knowing" something was amiss. She told her husband that she and Reham needed to see the doctor urgently—and alone. At that point, he shared the details of Reham's diagnosis.

Umm Reham did not know how to interpret the presence of an extra chromosome in her daughter's cells. "[I] thought 'Oh, it's better?! Maybe she will be a genius!'" Her husband countered this interpretation. "This extra chromosome . . . it damages. It doesn't make things better." His description of "damage" reflects the power of a medical model of disability that foregrounds the cognitive impairment and health issues resulting from trisomy 21. But for Umm Reham, a college-educated woman who planned to become a stay-at-home mom, damage assumed a different and more menacing form. An acquaintance in her extended social circle had given birth to a baby with Down syndrome around the same time, yet the aftershocks of this event led to dramatically dissimilar outcomes. "They're divorced!" Umm Reham exclaimed. "As soon as the girl was born, when the mother returned home after the hospital, the lock on the door was changed. 'Go to your family,' [her husband said]."

The lurking specter of Jordan's patriarchal legal system abruptly reappeared in this grim counterpoint through the mechanism of guardianship. Umm Reham continued, telling me that "the daughter died. Very recently. She got sick, and they couldn't afford to take her to a hospital where she could get direct ICU care. She died on the hospital bed. The hospital refused to release the body to her mother [a consequence of the legal powers vested in men as guardians]. They insisted on waiting for her father, who had been wholly uninvolved in her life up until its premature ending. Eventually, his family showed up to claim the body and pay the expenses. They dealt with the burial, and the mother had no say." After dwelling momentarily on this heartbreaking chain of events, Umm Reham returned to her own much happier story and reaffirmed, "There are different reactions. But no, my husband, he loves Reham very much, and his family, and my family. Everyone."

Exclusionary communication between doctors and husbands clearly endangered women and children by giving husbands time to "change the lock on the door," to quote Umm Reham.[19] Other mothers, however, faced a problem of overly collective communication. Rather than first discussing their son's Down syndrome privately, Umm Abud's doctor announced that Abud was "mongholi" in front of extended family members who had gathered to meet the new baby. "It should have been between us, in the office," she exclaimed, the tone of her voice conveying dismay and still raw emotion. Her husband was furious about Abud's diagnosis, and he initially wanted a divorce. While their marriage survived this turbulent period, members of their extended and immediate family distanced themselves from Umm Abud and her son. Even her older children, Abud's own siblings, could not understand why their mother decided to "keep" their youngest brother, implying that she should have institutionalized him in a residential center.

Women repeatedly affirmed that the birth of a baby with Down syndrome could lead to divorce. In such cases, patriarchy and patriliny converged to assign mothers outsized responsibility for the gestational process, both through and beyond biogenetic frameworks of fertilization and fetal development. While the moral consensus around this outcome continues to shift, they still took the risk seriously. Allowing for some exceptions, divorce is considered a socially damaging process that disproportionately harms women and children. Yet people also readily acknowledged that a preponderance of factors could contribute to unexpected birth outcomes, from medical error or paternally inherited conditions to acts of God. A man who chose to abandon his wife and disabled child, moreover, would undoubtedly receive criticism, perhaps to his face and most certainly behind his back, for failing to live up to the masculine ideals of protecting and providing for one's family.

Biomedicine privileged husbands' authority (also reinforced by guardianship), and some men leveraged this power against their wives and children.[20] But it was not the only possible outcome, nor is it the only possible interpretation for the selective communication that some of my interlocutors experienced. In getting to know Umm Reham and her family, I came to see her husband's delay as an attempt to protect his wife from the suspicion that she would face disproportionately, whether from their immediate family or their wider social networks. After all, he called *her* mother, not his, after learning about their daughter's condition. While misaligned with a normative bioethical prioritization of patient autonomy, it is not unusual for families in Jordan to withhold diagnostic and prognostic information from loved ones as protection against shock, which they consider an additional and serious risk to health and recovery (Arabiat et al. 2011; Dasoqi et al. 2013).

Down syndrome, to be clear, is not an illness from which one "recovers." But in the early moments with a new baby and a diagnosis that carried unclear implications for the future, the specificities of Down syndrome mattered less than its outsized social impacts, which parents bore unequally. The divergent outcomes of selective communication, however, left women more vulnerable to their relationships with spouses, which were rarely unconnected from each spouse's relationships with their own natal kin.

MARRIAGE AND MODERNNESS

Disability-focused research in the fields of rehabilitation and psychology shows considerable interest in the impact that childhood disability, and Down syndrome in particular, has on marital and family cohesion. The time I spent with families led me to approach this question from the opposite direction. Rather than ask how Down syndrome affects marriage, I came to appreciate how marriage in Jordan participates in making Down syndrome. Distancing oneself or one's family from a relative with Down syndrome reveals a disability world in which actors take connectivity between kin for granted and where designations of "normal"—or not—are distributed among kin and potential kin (Joseph 1993).[21] Marriage mediates these connections, even as the practices and meanings associated with marriage continue to change in ways that reflect broader socioeconomic and political shifts (Adely 2016; Hughes 2021; MacDougall 2021). Neither extant nor emergent moral rubrics countered marriage's role in legitimating relations and marking a boundary of adulthood. Nor did people strive to radically alter how heritability contributed to constructions of self and relatedness. Instead, families assembled and reconfigured moral rubrics of medicine, religion, and human rights to incorporate Down syndrome into kinship futures.

Hana (introduced above), who told me about the television interviews while reflecting on the contested link between Down syndrome and heritability, stressed that despite some immediate shock, her parents and the rest of their family quickly accepted Jamal's Down syndrome. Her parents concentrated their postdiagnosis efforts on locating services and acquiring more information. When we met, Jamal was in his early twenties, so their family belonged to the pre-CRPD generation defined by fewer health and social services. Most of their kin welcomed Jamal into their lives, although a small minority had chosen to distance themselves. (Months later, I accompanied participants in an outing Jamal attended, which was organized by the Al-Nur Society. As the group trudged single file along a grassy section of Amman's less developed northern edge, a large white SUV pulled over to the side of the road. The chaperones tensed as the car slowed down but quickly relaxed as the driver began to excitedly call out greetings to Jamal, his nephew, and whipped out his smartphone to record their encounter. Jamal, meanwhile, excitedly repeated, "My uncle! That's my uncle!" They waved and called out mutual wishes for good health and safe travels.)

The problem, Hana explained, was that too many families still felt *haraj* and *thaqafat al-ʿayb* (embarrassment and a culture of shame). This led them to believe they could not leave the house—or be seen—with a child with Down syndrome. Much of our conversation pivoted around *ʿayb*. This term once preoccupied anthropologists involved in debating the existence of a so-called honor and shame complex across the region, but more recent generations of anthropologists have turned decisively away from engaging with these categories.[22] While *ʿayb* literally translates to "defect," its "colloquial use pertains to behaviours that are considered disgraceful or inappropriate" (Odgaard 2022, 39). *ʿAyb* offers a relatively uncontroversial moral rubric, even as its component parts are dynamic and open to debate. The term signals boundaries and designates breaches of social norms positioned at the intersections of gender, sexuality, age, and class.[23]

Hana refused to feel *haraj* and *ʿayb* by claiming her positionality as a modern, educated woman. In doing so, she employed aspects of the disability imaginaries outlined in chapter 2. Recently, she had heard about the father of a three-year-old with Down syndrome who wanted to divorce his wife and remarry to have "normal" children. "Can you imagine?!" she exclaimed. "We're in 2015, and there are still people who think like this!" For Hana, this man's reaction was not merely immoral; it was regressive. He had failed to cultivate a modern—and thus moral—rubric appropriate for the year 2015. To contextualize families' variable reactions to the birth of a disabled child, she offered me the saying that "not all fingers on the hand are the same." Some families felt they could not present a child with Down syndrome to their larger kin and social networks and "hid" them at home. Others considered this behavior and justifications for it as profoundly misguided. Those in the latter camp *also* mobilized 'ayb to designate disability-related stigma as itself backwardness, recasting the purported link between Down syndrome and moral hazard as the actual problem.

In conjunction with disability, 'ayb designated social risk and enacted moral censure, but my interlocutors worked to redirect its logics and targets by reconfiguring moral rubrics available to them. Hana, for example, inverted dominant norms on their own terms. She could not recall Jamal's Down syndrome affecting their older brother's marital pursuits, but when she came of age, she acknowledged that "some people that came to ask for my hand, and when they knew that I had a mongholi brother they distanced themselves. . . . So, some people said, 'Don't let Jamal enter [the room]; that way people can't see him.' I said to them, 'On the contrary, from the first day they will see him. Anyone who wants to marry me needs to see him. And anyone who doesn't like him. . . . See you later! Allah ma'ak!'" (God be with you/bye!). Flipping the script, Hana assessed the potential of *her* suitors, and *their* families, based on how they treated Jamal; he became an asset and not the liability. She was not the only young woman I met who used similar encounters to assess the suitability of potential suitor. The ability to make such claims and translate them into practice, however, required material and symbolic power, not to mention support from parents, siblings (especially brothers), and larger social networks.

Across distinctions of class and religiosity, families worked to remake Down syndrome through shared and modified moral rubrics. Marshaling the social and cultural capital at their disposal, they reframed associations between Down syndrome and 'ayb as evidence of weakness, casting the accusation back on the accuser. Hana did this by claiming Jamal's value for screening potential suitors and by dismissing fears about heritability as scientifically unsound. Some women, however, reproduced a broader framework of blame while refusing the specific charge of maternal accountability.

MOTHERS AND MOTHERS-IN-LAW

Umm May and her husband settled in Amman after fleeing worsening violence in Iraq, sacrificing their previously middle-class life in the hopes of building a more stable kinship future. Immobilized by political uncertainty and complicated border regimes, they struggled with the financial and procedural barriers that affect all but the most privileged passport holders in Jordan. Because of the downward class mobility their displacement precipitated (Twigt 2022), Umm May found herself co-residing with her husband's parents and unmarried sister out of necessity. During my first visit to their home, located in one of the most economically depressed neighborhoods of East Amman, Umm May's sisters-in-law, nephews, and nieces gathered to share a family lunch in the apartment's dark and somewhat cramped quarters. My field notes from this visit reflect my confusion, as I tried to keep track of everyone's names and ascertain who was related to whom and how.

When I asked about how Umm May coped with the shock of May's diagnosis, Umm May's sisters-in-law responded with a chorus of rebuttals. "No, no no! There was no shock!" From the kitchen, Umm May shouted in agreement. "There was no shock, Christine!" Alia, the sister-in-law who appointed herself as Umm May's representative and my official guide to their neighborhood, further elaborated on the problem with my question. Shock, she explained, was not something a Muslim should feel about the arrival of a child with a disability. "Everything is a gift from God. There was no shock, because why would we be shocked by what God has given us?" My question about shock lingered for both women, as I would later learn. But during this initial visit to their home, Umm May's sisters-in-law steered our conversation.

When Umm May and her husband began to recover from the financial havoc of displacement, they decided it was time to move. I visited her after they were well settled into their new space, almost a year later. The bright and airy apartment was located up one flight of stairs, a welcome change from their previously ground-floor, partially subterranean accommodations. It offered their five children more space to play and study, and it boasted the additional advantage of being in a different neighborhood from Umm May's in-laws. Running around to prepare the lunch her children would expect on the table when they returned from school, Umm May appeared significantly more at ease, despite the strain that their relocation placed on their relationship with her husband's kin. She also shared an ambivalent narrative about May's birth, reflecting more candidly on the questions of shock, faith, and responsibility that May's Down syndrome precipitated.

Umm May's family had become part of a global Iraqi diaspora (Saleh 2020). She had not seem them for over a decade, and she missed them terribly. While they stayed connected through family WhatsApp chats, she held little hope that they would all be physically reunited during her parents' lifetimes. Initially grasping for the right words, she described them as more open-minded than her husband's family. She recalled a terrible fight they had after her mother-in-law criticized Umm May's eldest daughter for dressing "inappropriately" and strenuously objected to the teenager's use of makeup. Umm May considered her daughter's experimentation with fashion and cosmetics as perfectly normal, and she was not concerned. This was but one example of how class backgrounds and worldviews shaped divergent approaches to the dynamic and often fraught standards of moral, modern Muslim womanhood (see also Adely 2012b; MacDougall 2019, 2021).

Without her sisters-in-law present, Umm May no longer negated the shock that she felt after May's diagnosis. In the beginning, she did not understand what Down syndrome meant. She worried about May's safety and about their futures. Raising a child with Down syndrome while navigating the unpredictable economic, infrastructural, and political conditions of displacement required more work and time than she had available. Umm May tried to enroll May in preschool, but several directors turned them away under the pretense that they were not equipped to meet May's needs. She knew that she could fight their refusals, which were technically illegal even under the older disability rights law in effect during my fieldwork. But she could not take on what would surely become a time-consuming campaign while also caring for her other children and contending with the financial and practical constraints that limited her capacity to move through the city.

The situation made her feel deeply guilty, but Umm May never entertained the possibility that *she* might be responsible for May's Down syndrome. After all, she reasoned, half-laughing, she and her husband's families were not even from the same country! They were not "relatives," unlike so many of the Jordanians they met (I will return to this comment in the next section).[24] Umm May did not specify that a lack of shared genes defined the "distance" in their marriage, but her comment reflects widespread awareness that marriage between relatives can lead to health problems. Dismissing the possibility that she had contributed to May's Down syndrome, Umm May instead hypothesized that the constant stress of living with her mother-in-law affected May's development in utero. Her interpretation shows that women could reproduce gendered logics of heritability and blame even as they rerouted the accusations typically leveled against them toward other women in their lives. This involved shifting from a lineal reckoning of heritability to more diffuse notions about the womb and the importance of creating a healthy environment for pregnancy.

Umm May felt that her affines overstepped their boundaries and undermined her parental authority. She reminded me of my first visit to their old home, expressing incredulity that *they* had felt entitled to respond to my questions about raising a child with Down syndrome. A sense of parenting as shared labor, however, is not wholly atypical in Jordan. Aunts, uncles, and even cousins often play significant roles in the lives of nieces, nephews, and younger cousins, blurring the lines between kin statuses and roles. While Umm May felt mistreated by her affinal kin, her relationship with her husband afforded her strength. They were partners who weathered profound geopolitical turmoil and trauma, and they held great warmth and affection for each other and for their children. Marriage brought conflict and tension into Umm May's world in the form of affinal kin, but it also brought a life companion, love, support, and motherhood.

May herself embodied this paradox; the tensions between her mother and her paternal grandparents did not spill over into her life. Instead, her father's kin doted on the joyous, raucous toddler, whose smile and giggles lit up the room, her dark ringlets constantly shaking with laughter from all the things she found amusing and worthy of attention. Not all children had access to a home like hers, which was filled with warmth, stimulation, and learning, despite the ongoing intergenerational drama. The rich sensory and social input that her family provided offset her limited participation in the early intervention services that I examine in chapter 4. It was simply too difficult for the family to arrange or afford the transportation costs required for consistent attendance. Yet May had already begun to encounter institutional barriers that her family had a limited capacity to manage, and missed opportunities in early childhood could have "cascading" effects over time (Manderson and Warren 2016).

Umm May's narrative attests to how moral rubrics available for making Down syndrome remained steeped in dominant logics of kinship and gender. Like Umm Reham, Umm May counted her husband as an ally, a friend, and a devoted father. And like Hana and Umm Munir, Umm May drew on diffuse scientific knowledge around consanguinity to point out that she and her husband were neither close nor even distant kin. On a deeper level, however, her framing still positioned Down syndrome as the outcome of relations that had somehow "gone wrong." In hypothesizing about her mother-in-law's role, she embraced the porous sociality and embodied relationality that contribute to fears about heritability. In the privacy of her own home, Umm May affirmed her experience of shock. She did not, however, equate shock with a lack of faith in God, which was something that she—like many of my interlocutors—possessed in abundance.

A NONSECULAR GENEALOGY

Umm Sami and I met during my first months of fieldwork, when she and her son Sami worked the table at a charitable bazaar located inside a popular mall, displaying handicrafts produced by members of the Al-Nur Society's youth group. We later reconnected at the same Ramadan iftar where I sat with Umm Zayna. While I thought Umm Sami looked familiar, I could not initially place her. Dressed in her customary black jilbab and hijab, she stood chatting quietly with Umm Karim, who had brought her son Karim to the gathering, as well as his older sister and their new baby brother. Petite and soft-spoken, Umm Karim hovered on the edge of the party's activities while nervously guarding her youngest son in her arms. The overtures of the other children—all of whom delighted in the presence of a baby—made her uneasy. When I went to greet Umm Karim and offer my congratulations, I mentioned the possibility of conducting an interview, which we had discussed when she and her mother-in-law had attended an early intervention session a few months prior. At that point, Umm Sami interjected and asked, "Well, do you want to talk to *me*?!"

Initially confused, I tilted my head somewhat hesitantly. Umm Sami clarified that she was Sami's mom and pointed him out in the crowd. With the light bulb switched on, we exchanged numbers and confirmed with a successfully initiated WhatsApp thread. A few weeks later, I arrived at the apartment building Sami and his family called home. My taxi driver was intrigued by my thoroughly working-class destination in a neighborhood known for industrial workshops and a large community of displaced Syrians. He then gave me a second probing glance when he saw Sami waiting to escort me inside. After greeting Umm Sami with the appropriate cheek kisses and inquiries as to our health and families, we went through the customary consumption of coffee, food, and tea before starting a more formal interview.

Sami's diagnosis came unexpectedly in a hospital emergency room. The doctors had already informed her husband that Sami had Down syndrome, but they initially told Umm Sami only that he was "sick." When the new parents returned some weeks later because Sami had fallen ill, an unfamiliar doctor saw him and asked, "Who is that? The *mongholi* child?" Umm Sami was taken aback. "I asked him what *mongholi* meant, and he told me it means that the child is disabled. And he apologized a lot, but I was very angry. I told him, 'Alhamdulillah, he is from God.'" The idea that disability and illness constitute punishments from God reappeared in conversations with non-Jordanians, as well as with Jordanians who distanced themselves from what they described as "popular" religious beliefs. Yet none of my interlocutors suggested as much. Instead, they incorporated Islam as a critical moral rubric for making Down syndrome. They rejected the notion that disability represented a "curse" because such an interpretation grossly mischaracterizes God's relationship with human beings and ignores His essential qualities of mercy and generosity. "God does not send one life to punish another," one mother explained by way of succinctly dismissing this claim.

Families mobilized Islamic values of compassion and conviction to disrupt moral rubrics that stressed the importance of marriageability and family reputation, which they glossed as "cultural" in nature. It troubled them that the interpretation of Down syndrome as some form of divine punishment existed in their own community, whether they defined that locally or in terms of a global Muslim community (*ummah*). They felt especially frustrated when non-Muslims associated them with what they deemed a combination of religious ignorance and cultural backwardness. Nevertheless, their keen awareness and desire to refute this framework suggested that it maintained an uncomfortable presence in everyday landscapes of making Down syndrome. Refusing the doctor's attempt to define her son in terms of genetic alterity, Umm Sami instead located him in a genealogy shared by all humans; Sami was "from God." That was a truth no legitimate doctor could dispute. During our conversation, however, Umm Sami repeatedly decried the harmful gossip she endured at the hands of her husband's relatives and their neighbors. She wondered about the impact of heritability, as she and her husband were related, but she pointed to the presence of Down syndrome in parts of the world not known for practicing cousin marriage. If consanguinity were a significant contributing factor, why would the condition manifest globally?

Across the SWANA region, consanguineous marriages constitute between 20 to 50 percent of all marital unions; in Jordan, consanguineous marriage is declining but accounts for over one-quarter of all marriages (Islam 2021).[25] Accordingly, Jordan and other SWANA states, along with international development and health organizations, have prioritized research exploring the links between consanguinity and comorbidity. Consanguinity increases the risk for certain conditions and diseases, especially disorders with an autosomal recessive inheritance pattern. Existing research on Down syndrome has generated contradictory findings, and most trustworthy studies have found not yet found any evidence of a meaningful relationship between the two (Hamamy et al. 2011). Further complicating matters, established traditions of endogamy can increase the homozygosity of a gene pool and have an impact on community health profiles irrespective of marital consanguinity (Bittles 2005). These subtle complexities nevertheless tend to recede from global public health depictions of consanguinity and local renderings of the practice as well (Shaw and Raz 2015).

Not knowing why Sami was born with Down syndrome enabled Umm Sami to contest accusations that she and Abu Sami were somehow responsible; the eventual birth of their younger son without Down syndrome further amplified this productive uncertainty (Whitmarsh 2008). Sami's parents also benefited from the influence of a family friend who happened to be a nurse. Shortly after Sami's diagnosis, she advised them to remember that "[Sami] came to us like this from God and insha'allah; we will have children who are better than him. So we accepted him, and Abu Sami accepted it. And even three years later, he told me that if I got pregnant it would be fine, and even if I didn't, it would be okay. . . . I got pregnant with Jawwad. I was afraid, but I was praying that God would give me a brother or sister for Sami. And then I gave birth to Jawwad. This convinced our relatives that the reason [Sami has Down syndrome] was not because I was old or because my husband and I are related."

Umm Sami combined established facts and continued gaps in scientific knowledge with the foundational certainty that God does not make mistakes. The totality and completeness of God's wisdom offered a compelling mode of resisting stigma, especially when parallel accusations of scientific ignorance might otherwise fail to shift existing moral rubrics. Accepting that Down syndrome, like pregnancy itself, came from God, Umm and Abu Sami moved forward in their lives as a couple, as parents, and as a family. In addition to their joy over having another son, Umm Sami described a distinct sense of relief. She hoped that Jawwad would not only become Sami's friend and companion but also his eventual caregiver. I return to this point in chapter 6.

MORAL RUBRICS AND KINSHIP FUTURES

For Umm Zayna, diagnosis cast a shadow over the past while raising painful questions about kinship futures. Patriarchal and patrilineal influences on family security loomed large in her and many women's early fears about Down syndrome, which materialized through concrete, visceral matters of care. In shock, the unknowns of Down syndrome collided with the intimate realities of gendered blame that deemed mothers responsible for "abnormal" babies. For some women, divorce, rejection by in-laws, or estrangement from kin appeared as barely conceivable possibilities. Others, however, found themselves thrust into new and lifeworld-altering circumstances. Marriage and kinship created social hazards, but they also offered tools for cultivating new kinship futures and new ways of making Down syndrome. Many women emphasized the singularity of their relationships, as well as their personal qualities of ingenuity, tenacity, and faith, to process how having a child with Down syndrome could precipitate such manifestly different outcomes.

The moral rubrics that families deployed to make Down syndrome in the aftermath of diagnosis drew on dynamic and overlapping traditions, including biomedicine, Islam, education, and ideas about modernness (Deeb 2006). Gendered realities of childcare intersected with gendered ideologies of modernity to position mothers as key maintainers and innovators of these rubrics. Diagnosis, however, is only ever a beginning, and it is a partial one at that. As Zayna moved from infancy to early childhood, she would become a more active participant in the relational negotiations of care and circumstance that make Down syndrome. The future-oriented fears of that postdiagnosis moment did not disappear but transformed over time and amid expanding opportunities for therapeutic intervention and community building. In chapter 4, I examine how mothers became stewards and targets in Jordan's changing landscape of childhood disability.

4 · AMBIVALENT INTERVENTIONS

"Training for what?"

Shuruq lay on a fuzzy blanket in the room dedicated to early intervention consultations at Al-Nur Society. Many of the babies and toddlers I observed in similar circumstances would start grasping at the foam mat underneath. Its pastel components were designed to fit together like a puzzle, which provided growing bodyminds opportunities to work on grip strength and spatial reasoning (or to take exploratory nibbles). But Shuruq lay quietly on her back, with her mother and eldest sister kneeling beside her. Clearly lethargic, she wore a white spaghetti-strap tank top that had been repurposed into a dress, but it was still too large for her small frame. No older than eighteen months, Shuruq was recovering from a virus that had led to an inpatient stay at a private hospital. She had then acquired a secondary infection that left her frail. And yet, Umm Shuruq had arrived at Al-Nur eager to learn when she might begin training (*tadrib*) with her youngest daughter.

"Training for what?" asked Batool. The early intervention specialist gazed at Umm Shuruq with some concern. "She's sick, Umm Shuruq. She's weak. You need to wait for her to get stronger." Ultimately, Batool provided Umm Shuruq with basic "homework," directing her instructions more toward Shuruq's eldest sister, then in her late teens, than to Umm Shuruq herself. She encouraged both women to engage Shuruq with sounds and sights that would hold her attention—snapping, clapping, cooing her name at a high pitch, shaking a stuffed animal with bells attached at the ends. She also recommended that they redirect Shuruq's tendency to arrange her lower limbs in a "frog-leg" position, which could leave her underdeveloped muscles cramped and stiff if held for too long.[1] One possible technique involved gently tying a blanket around Shuruq's straightened legs, but only for short periods of time. Above all, however, Batool reiterated that Shuruq needed time to regain strength and recover from her illness.

After Umm Shuruq and her daughters departed, Batool expressed frustration with a degree of candor that took me by surprise. What, Batool wanted to know, did Umm Shuruq hope to achieve with an ill and underweight baby? She repeatedly referred to Shuruq as *meskina* (poor thing/girl), a term that also stood out to me. Parents and specialists, Batool included, usually avoided this language, which connoted pity and reproduced the unwelcome framing of Down syndrome as a tragedy or disaster. For Batool, however, Shuruq's evident poor health and Umm Shuruq's insensitivity to her daughter's vulnerable state justified this description. I viewed Umm Shuruq differently, interpreting her desire for training as a reflection of a entrepreneurial and proactive spirit encouraged by new therapeutic regimes. However prematurely, Umm Shuruq embraced a core message of early intervention—that therapeutic impacts during the critical window of early childhood cannot be replicated later in life.[2] Batool, however, remained unsettled by Umm Shuruq's pursuit.

Early intervention (*al-tadakhkhul al-mubakkir*) encompasses a constellation of physical, speech, and occupational therapies designed to address the needs of children experiencing or at risk for developmental delay and disability; children with Down syndrome are considered prime candidates.[3] These therapies amount to what anthropologist Eliza Williamson describes as "habilitative care" because they mobilize "a range of substances, technologies, and techniques understood to encourage maximum potential development of embodied abilities in young disabled children" (2024, 11). They are not *re*habilitative because they do not seek to restore lost function. Instead, they are oriented around normative benchmarks that a child has not yet met or is at risk of failing to meet (Friedner 2022a; Mauldin 2016; Williamson 2024).

In this chapter, I consider how early intervention engendered opportunities for connection and empowerment alongside new forms of exposure and scrutiny. These affordances and ambivalences were not confined to the bodyminds of children with Down syndrome. Instead, "multiple registers and temporalities of development" (Friedner 2015, 6) coalesced *in and between* children and their mothers (and a cadre of teachers and specialists), linking them at the nexus of personal, familial, and national projects of "embodied development" (Sargent 2019). While ostensibly focused on the potentiality of children with disabilities, early intervention invited mothers to embark on their own "projects of becoming" (Mattingly 2014a, 5; see also Friedner 2022b). They received these invitations cautiously, engaging or declining for various reasons and to various ends. The title of this chapter plays with the ambivalences that emerged through these regimes of habilitative care. In addition to intervention, *tadakhkhul* can also connote "meddling."[4]

The specific program that connected Umm Shuruq and Batool goes by the name of Portage, which refers to its origins in Portage, Wisconsin (Shearer and Shearer 1972). It first entered Southwest Asia and North Africa (SWANA) in 1984 via the Gaza Strip (Faour et al. 2006), expanding as specialists worked to address acute impacts of the First Intifada and broader consequences of Palestinian childhood under Occupation (Oakland 1997).[5] The Arab Council for Child-hood Development then adopted the model and began implementing training sessions across the region, in collaboration with governmental and international partners (Faour et al. 2006; Hadidi and Al Khateeb 2015). Although its efficacy remains debated (Al-Wedyan and Al-Oweidi 2021; Brue and Oakland 2001; Cameron 2021), the program offers a low-tech, low-cost approach to early inter-vention that utilizes household objects and everyday routines as therapeutic opportunities.

Portage relies on parents—and given the gendered realities of childcare, mothers are typically primary facilitators—to track their child's progress across five developmental areas: communication and literacy, social-emotional devel-opment, exploration and approaches to learning, purposeful motor activity, and sensory organization (Barakat et al. 2004; CESA5 2023; Sarouphim and Kassem 2022).[6] In its most typical configuration, a teacher or visitor meets with a parent (usually the mother) and child in their home and conducts an initial assessment using Portage's extensive skills-based checklist.[7] This informs the child's individ-ualized learning plan, which parents implement using activity cards designed to target priority skills across the aforementioned areas. Ideally, visits with a Por-tage teacher or facilitator occur at weekly intervals. Parents and teachers gather observational data, create weekly plans, and document yearly assessments with materials provided in the Portage tool kit. While Portage focuses on early child-hood development, the program stresses the formative influence of the parent-child relationship and the habilitative potentiality of both children and parents.

From its Wisconsin origins, Jordanian enactments of Portage materialized through the broader disability imaginaries outlined in chapter 2, guiding fami-lies' engagements with its habilitative logics. In the next section, I explore how these imaginaries situated governmental and institutional support for early intervention as evidence of Jordan's commitment to disability rights. This fram-ing turned parental compliance into an index of their commitment to inclusion and acceptance.[8] I then explore the gendered and maternal interventions that early intervention catalyzed, which compelled mothers to navigate expectations for "good" motherhood and "good" womanhood through the pursuit of children's embodied development. Finally, I examine how childhood disability became a site for interworldly interventions (Friedner 2019, 2020).[9] While families readily incorporated secular framings of disability into their everyday practices of mak-ing Down syndrome, they also took seriously—and took comfort in—the irre-futable truth that God does not make mistakes. Keenly interested in maximizing habilitative outcomes, they also cultivated acceptance of God's wisdom to paro-chialize the normalizing contradictions of habilitative therapies. While decidedly ambivalent, a sense of opportunity permeated these sites and modes of interven-tion, making early childhood a period of expanding possibility and intensifying pressure.

INTERVENTION'S IMAGINARIES

Pursuing early intervention opened women up to judgment while failing to take advantage of early intervention precipitated the same. The criticisms they faced and reproduced drew on the grammar of "culturalism" (Sukarieh 2012, 2016; see chapter 2) that infuses Jordan's broader disability imaginaries. When Umm Shuruq arrived at Al-Nur with a sick and tired baby, she wanted to affirm her acceptance of Shuruq's Down syndrome and her commitment to supporting her daughter's needs. These efforts demonstrated her refusal to hide Shuruq at home or abandon her to a residential center. The latter exemplified rejection (*rafad*), or the lack of parental investment that betrayed indifference to a child's possible futures. When a family rejected disability, was it a symptom or a cause of society's rejection? People answered the question differently, but they adhered to the terms of the underlying interpretive framework. This imaginary plotted Jordan on a developmental trajectory where it moved closer—but not close enough—to acceptance, while manifestations (or accusations) of rejection mapped onto existing social fault lines.

Families from "the governorates" (which colloquially referred to any of the eleven governorates outside Amman) and from East Amman were perceived as more likely to reject disability. This marked them as in greater need of intervention, early and otherwise. After one of my first visits to the eastern neighborhood of Jabal Ahmar, Batool could not contain her curiosity about my impressions of the city's "other half." Westerners do not typically visit Amman's working-class and economically distressed areas. But for that matter, neither did Batool. Like many Ammanis, her movements around the city were tightly linked to her family's home and the neighborhoods she frequented for work and school. Other areas remained largely unfamiliar to her. That a six-mile drive from one end of Amman to the other could take fifteen minutes or sixty, depending on the time of day and day of the week, reinforced these constrained geographies of circulation.

During my visit to Jabal Ahmar, I met a young girl with vision impairment who lived next door to the family hosting me for lunch. She navigated around the space of her neighbors' small, narrow house largely by touch and managed quite well, but the same strategy did not serve her in school. She was falling behind her peers and would likely need to repeat a grade. As I shared this scenario with Batool, she grew increasingly upset. "They need to go to the Ministry [of Social Development]! The thing with people in places like Jabal Ahmar is that they complain about how hard things are and how there's nothing for them. There is. Things are not as bad as they say. Blind children can go to school! Things are not that bad, Christine!"

At some point during this spirited missive, Batool's co-worker Kawthar walked into the room. "Kawthar," Batool instructed, "explain to Christine what families in East Amman are like." Kawthar turned and shrugged. "They just want someone to find them a center where they can deposit their kids, and that's it." These stereotypes contradicted the nuanced analyses that Batool and Kawthar shared with me on other occasions. Both women were quite sensitive to how class and cultural politics obfuscate the challenges of raising a disabled child in Jordan, drawing from their careers as special educators and their identities as born-and-raised Ammanis of Palestinian descent. The availability and ease with which they nevertheless fell into such tropes attests to the force of a disability imaginary that bluntly slots acceptance and rejection into familiar fault lines of class, ethnicity, education, and piety, even for women well versed in living the complexities of their intersections.

Practically speaking, families in East Amman faced significantly longer commutes to access the services predominantly located in central and West Amman, which increased their likelihood of missing appointments or failing to show up for events. This reinforced a narrative that poorer families were less dedicated to their children and less willing or capable of undertaking the work that acceptance required. Despite widespread recognition that government inefficiency and a lack of accessible transportation generate serious challenges for most disabled Jordanians and their families, activists, specialists, and families themselves often described rejection as a primarily *cultural* problem. Some families and individuals did struggle with acceptance (whether they vocalized this or not), but accusations of rejection mirrored the culturalism that similarly drives accusations of hiding, recasting structural barriers in terms of moral lack and cultural malaise.

When pressed, however, most women offered more nuanced interpretations of how class and privilege shaped the terrain of acceptance and rejection. Some highlighted poor, "good" families who accepted their child's disability and contrasted them with wealthy, "bad" families who rejected their child. Reem, a special educator who offered tutorials and support services to families, lived in and primarily served fellow residents of her thoroughly working-class neighborhood in East Amman. But her professional experience took her all over the city. She had worked in public school and private school resource rooms, as well as at special education centers, before eventually moving into more senior administrative roles. Responding to my questions about acceptance, she shared the following example: "I used to work at a center near [an embassy on Zahran street]. They wouldn't even write this one child's name out because his family didn't want it known. He was listed on his chart as 'S.' These people are so 'sophisticated,' and they don't want anyone to know about the child! Here in East Amman, people are different. They're more open. They want to help and are more helpful." Reem inverted Batool and Kawthar's argument by suggesting that in West Amman, while people were more likely to possess the capital needed to access high-quality services, they also proved more sensitive to the possibility that disability might damage the family reputation. Affluence, according to Reem, not poverty, intensified stigma and led certain families to struggle with acceptance.

Hiding certainly seemed easier to do in the well-built, spacious high rises or villas found in West Amman, where people were less likely to know their neighbors or interact with them; where the wide, smooth streets lacked pedestrians, and nonfunctional sidewalks hovered at perilously high altitudes; where homeowners planted palm trees in the middle of existing walkways to dissuade overflow parking. East Amman's more cramped and deteriorated living conditions meant that domestic life spilled over into the streets and onto the rooftops. This made intimacy among neighbors more inevitable and mundane, whether one desired it or not. Ultimately, people offered divergent interpretations of what acceptance looked like and why rejection persisted, but they adhered to the core poles of this imaginary. Within the habilitative framework of early intervention, however, the clarity of acceptance became even more difficult to ascertain.

INTERVENTION INTO WHAT?

After the shock of diagnosis, as families settled into the rhythms of life as a Down syndrome family, they began attuning to the fleshy specificities of embodied difference and found themselves asking: What does it truly mean to accept this? The question reappeared throughout their lifelong struggles to cultivate kinship futures that included children with Down syndrome. As mothers acquired proficiency in the rhythms and formats of Portage (or other early intervention programs), they struggled with the paradoxes of habilitative care. The "successes" and "failures" that they encountered while pursuing benchmarks of embodied development prompted critical reflection. How *should* they balance the potentiality of bodily plasticity against the fleshy and sometimes unyielding realities of impairment? In other words, "by investing so much time, money, and labor in the habilitation of their children, were parents not cleaving to the idea that the more typical or 'normate' [Garland-Thomson 1997] their children could become, the better?" (Williamson 2024, 11).

Early intervention unsettled the binary of acceptance-and-rejection, instead amplifying the ambiguities of Down syndrome's "doubled discourse of sameness and difference" (Rapp 1999, 293). Was a child with Down syndrome *zayy ayy tifl tani* (like any other child)? Emphatically yes, in so many ways. But also no, in ways that felt equally critical to recognize and for which to create space. Bodies may be plastic and moldable, but they also have limits. Muscles can be trained and strengthened, but how do such efforts interact with the higher dosage of collagen that results from an extra copy of chromosome 21 and affects muscle tone at the cellular and musculoskeletal levels (Dey et al. 2013; Foley and Killeen 2019)? Habilitation made bodies more accessible to modification and manipulation, but its gaze also reaffirmed the body's unpredictability. Parents were certain, however, that the developmental delays experienced by children with Down syndrome could lead to ostracism and mistreatment by peers and elders, especially given the importance of bodily control to age-based and gendered expectations of propriety.

Some impairments threatened to become more disabling than others. The mouth, for example, played a significant role in making Down syndrome into a marked difference and a territory of possibility. From material concerns about the volume and texture of the tongue, to its functional role in producing speech—and the attendant language ideologies of "speaking well"—the mouth became a focal point of ambivalent intervention. During a Portage training at Al-Nur, I watched Batool scoop up a skeptical young volunteer and coo them into temporary acquiescence so she could demonstrate massage techniques for facilitating blood flow to facial muscles and for alleviating dry skin. Fluttering her fingers in gentle upward strokes around the neck and cheeks of her attentive (and occasionally disgruntled) model, the audience of mostly mothers observed, asked questions, and took notes on pads of paper or stored the details of such exercises to memory. In another popular drill, a trainer instructed mothers to place a small piece of date—well stocked in any Jordanian household—at the corner of their toddler's mouth. To retrieve the tasty morsel, the child would have to extend and twist their tongue, providing beneficial exercise. A small chunk of carrot—also nutritious—could also achieve the same goal.

Interventions aimed at strengthening children's oral faculties responded to serious challenges with eating, swallowing, and digesting. Concerns about infant feeding and healthy growth are not unique to children with Down syndrome, but long-term health issues associated with trisomy 21 have an impact on cardiopulmonary, airway, and metabolic systems (Bull et al. 2022), which intensified parents' and practitioners' sense of urgency. The desire to intervene, however, extended beyond questions of health to those of aesthetic norms (Livingston 2008). Parents worried about their children's divergent appearances and whether they would be able to satisfy the standards of proper oral comportment. Because of a relatively smaller upper jaw, many children (and adults) with Down syndrome appear to have larger than typical tongues, and parents expressed pointed anxieties about the resulting tongue protrusion. To address this concern, trainers recommended administering the smallest drop of lemon juice as a gentle but bitter corrective. A light tap with a finger could also work. Through these everyday activities, mothers (and sisters, aunts, grandmothers) gained knowledge and perspectives that transformed their relationships to their children and peers.

Umm Khaled's youngest son no longer participated in early intervention at Al-Nur because he started receiving these services at school, but she still liked to stop by and visit with staff. She lived in the neighborhood, so we often crossed paths at the local falafel shop where I made a habit of stopping to purchase my favorite breakfast order before settling in for the day. On one such morning, Umm Khaled entered the reception room and launched at lightning speed into telling us about a recent encounter still weighing on her mind: "Last week, we went to Burgerz. The whole family went. This woman, she was staring at Khaled. Just staring. I knew it was about Khaled. So, she approached me. 'Down?' she asked. 'Yes,' I responded. 'He's Down.' The woman paused, and then burst out, 'How can you get him to be so clean? My daughter, everything falls out of her mouth. She drools! The food . . . we can't take her out!'" She paused for dramatic effect. "Can you imagine" (*takhayy-ali*)?! That this stranger readily admitted to denying her daughter the opportunity to eat in a restaurant with the rest of her family left Umm Khaled deeply disturbed. Yet she also felt proud, and not only of Khaled, who was still considered significantly behind in meeting his own projected developmental milestones. Khaled's technical "success," from this stranger's perspective, validated Umm Khaled's efforts and their entire family's efforts by extension. At the same time, it served as a reminder of people's continued failure to accept her son or children like him.

Umm Khaled's experience echoed a story that Hana, introduced in chapter 3, shared with me about her brother Jamal. While walking together through a park near their home, Hana and Jamal ran into one of Hana's friends and stopped to chat. Eyeing Jamal, her friend asked whether they were related. Given what she perceived to be their obvious sibling resemblance, Hana found the question odd. Nevertheless, she confirmed that Jamal was her brother, at which point her friend confessed that she had a sister with Down syndrome. Their family did not include her sister in group outings because she walked too slowly and made a mess while eating, which included drooling or letting food fall from her mouth. Hana was appalled. She explained to me that everyone in her family worked with Jamal to ensure he could "eat properly," and Jamal himself eagerly embraced the work. Did he always achieve 100 percent success? Maybe not. But his efforts were good enough for them.

Both Hana's and Umm Khaled's encounters attested to their families' investments in habilitative care, but they also served as a painful reminder that misconceptions and discrimination led some families to neglect their kin. For them, this amounted to abandoning their responsibility, as Down syndrome families, to create greater acceptance in their society. Despite Jamal (Hana's brother) and Khaled (Umm Khaled's son) being over fifteen years apart in age, their participation in Portage shaped both families' experiences with making Down syndrome in early childhood. Yet early intervention also overlapped and resonated with an existing repertoire of pedagogical traditions that likewise strive to cultivate "normal" bodyminds.

PEDAGOGIES OF INTERVENTION

Mothers and special educators often encouraged each other with a reminder that "a mother is their child's first trainer" (*mudarrib*). This phrase echoed Umm

Shuruq's earnest request that Batool provide exercises to practice with Shuruq at home, which she described as training. Both words—"trainer" (*mudarrib*) and "training" (*tadrib*)—stem from the verb *darrab* (from the root form "darab"), which aligns with meanings of "to habituate to, become accustomed to, to practice, to drill, or train" (Wehr 1993). The pervasiveness of darrab gestured to a plurality of pedagogies that focused on cultivating children's bodyminds. Working across these different genealogies of intervention, parents consistently prioritized social proficiencies of speech and communication with a concomitant emphasis on training the mouth and its constitutive parts.[10]

Portage's interactional and quotidian intimacies gave teachers and experienced mothers a chance to reach more vulnerable peers as they grappled with the aftershocks of diagnosis (see chapter 3). But programs like Portage did not necessarily introduce radically new frameworks for conceptualizing or actualizing the potentiality of childhood. Instead, they widened the parameters of existing approaches to *tarbiyya* (pedagogy) and *adab* (etiquette). These terms encompass "a complex of valued dispositions (intellectual, moral, and social), appropriate norms of behavior, comportment, and bodily habitus" (El Shakry 1998, 127).[11] Writing about embodied pedagogies in the context of urban Cairo, for example, the anthropologist Farha Ghannam outlines an explicitly developmental logic:

> Children are instructed firmly and repeatedly about appropriate behavior and the importance of keeping their clothes clean during an outing. Such preparations teach children about proper bodily presentation and emphasize that how one appears can be even more important than personal comfort. Young boys and girls learn to endure the discomfort of tight shoes or a heavy jacket when these items match the rest of their outfit or are the only nice clothes available. As children become young adults, they increasingly become active in the management and regulation of their bodily comportment and representation. (2011, 791)

When read through the lens of disability, Ghannam's description raises certain questions: What happens to children who fail to meet normative standards of comportment and representation? What happens to children who *cannot* meet these standards? Programs nested under the umbrella of "early intervention" attest to the unpredictability and funkiness of actual bodyminds that may not easily accommodate smooth habituation into adult dispositions. But they also mark nonnormative bodyminds as worthy of investment and as capable of being molded.

Developmental delay and childhood disability are by no means radically novel expressions of the human condition. Nor are the solutions now offered through Portage and other habilitative therapies. My conversations with a lively septuagenarian named Umm Ali demonstrated some of these continuities of intervention. When I visited Umm Ali at her family home (her adult sons lived with their wives and children on separate floors above the ground floor that she shared with her husband and Ali), we spent a good amount of time relaxing on the covered patio outside. The sunny spring weather nurtured the home's green scaffolding, an effect largely achieved by the presence of grapevines that snaked their way across trellised woodwork. While busy preparing our lunch, Umm Ali's daughter-in-law also entered the discussion at various points to offer her perspective, and her own young daughter arrived home from primary school in time for our shared meal, eyeing me shyly with equal parts interest and skepticism.

A grandmotherly figure, Umm Ali repeatedly stressed how much had changed for families raising a child with Down syndrome in Jordan. Because Ali, her youngest son, was already in his late twenties when I met their family, she often lamented the lack of awareness and service provision that had shaped his childhood. Umm Ali received Ali's diagnosis after giving birth and while still in the hospital; her doctors quickly warned her that Ali would likely die during infancy. Disturbed by their lack of compassion and grim prognosis, she left almost immediately and began a lifelong quest for knowledge and supportive care. Some of the doctors she consulted suggested medicating Ali (she did not specify which medicines or what they were supposed to address), but Umm Ali felt that her best options lay outside biomedicine.

She devised and implemented a therapeutic program that bore a striking resemblance to elements of the early intervention and speech therapy regimens now offered to new mothers. "I knew I needed to do things with him, and I knew that first of all, I had to get him on a better eating schedule, and I had to do exercises with him." She made him a special barley soup.[12] She played sports with him to develop his strength and cardiovascular capacity. She used chewing gum to develop his oral and facial muscles. And she protected his vulnerable immune system by keeping him away from large crowds. She recalled that "I would always try to work on his speech at home, to the extent I could, because there were no speech therapists. . . . I would bring a mirror and teach him. I would ask, 'Did you see how [to say this]?' And I would slowly enunciate the letters. I would tell him that he has to exercise always so that his muscles get stronger. *When you speak well, people will accept you.* Drool would run down from his mouth because his muscles are weak. Alhamdulillah he stopped drooling, and he started to speak correctly, but it took a long time." Umm Ali considered Ali's relatively strong communication skills to be a product of their shared labor. Her efforts to work with her son, despite a lack of formal guidance by experts, attest to established traditions of cultivating embodied development.

By linking "speaking well" to acceptance, Umm Ali clarified social and relational dimensions of the latter. While language is central to personhood, the importance of speaking *well* highlights the more subtle barriers to acceptance faced by those who deviate from norms. As a nonnative Arabic speaker, I was occasionally struck by how expectations around "speaking well" created moments of shared experience between myself and companions with Down syndrome. While more formal acquaintances would kindly compliment my Arabic, those with whom I had a closer (and thus more frank) relationship teased me about my "heavy tongue" and strange grammatical contortions. Spending time around children and adults with a spectrum of speech impairments, I was surprised when native-Arabic speakers sometimes asked me to interpret their divergent styles of articulation. Occasionally, my field notes conveyed my frustration with the degree of noncomprehension exhibited by people without Down syndrome. They seemed unwilling to adapt and instead adhered to what Arseli Dokumacı describes as a "habitus of ableism" (2023). If I could understand my companions with speech impairments, native speakers around me most certainly could as well, if they tried. The sense of puzzlement—and consternation—encountered by those guilty of speaking "less than well" attests to how social norms differentially "define particular attributes as impairments" (Minich 2016); those affecting speech became more stigmatized and thus more disabling.[13]

Intervention for Whom?

During early childhood, many mothers described feeling a constant, sometimes agonizing sense of anxiety about their child's well-being and possible future. This stemmed in part from a medicalized framing of "early childhood" as the formative stage responsible for "determining" a child's future degree of disability. And as mechanisms for therapeutic surveillance expanded, women faced heightened scrutiny of their choices, their character, and their relationships. Seeking out opportunities to care for and advocate for their child, they found themselves engaging with kin and nonkin in unanticipated and unfamiliar ways, exposing themselves and their families to judgment. Locating (or being located by) Down syndrome and other disability-centered social networks, mothers became subjects of interventions alongside their children.

The relationships women forged in these new circumstances could be quite fragile, as they deliberated about whom they could trust and to what extent.[14] The anthropologist Cheryl Mattingly writes that "parents' ability to respond to the call or needs of their vulnerable children, and to create a social world in which their children can be better cared for, become primary moral projects . . . that change shape over time, requiring the development of communities of care" (2014a, 5). This description captures the intimate—and sometimes charged—relationships that women developed as they participated in communities driven by therapeutics or advocacy. In the tensions that surfaced between them, debates about "good" motherhood became a medium for enacting and embodying competing visions of progress and "modernity" (Abu-Lughod 1998; Adely 2009,

2012a; Deeb 2006; El Shakry 1998). These often crystallized in discussions about cultivating appropriate emotions and sensibilities.

Umm Fadi lived with her husband and their twenty-year-old son Fadi, the youngest of three children, in an affluent neighborhood of western Amman. While ostensibly at Al-Nur to pick up Fadi after youth club, she lingered one day to chat with Umm Adil and her oldest daughter Lamia, who often accompanied her mother and Adil to his sessions. Umm Adil was frustrated with Adil's continued lack of speech and what she perceived as his overall lack of progress since beginning early intervention and speech therapy. Drawing on her own lived expertise, Umm Fadi offered that when she needed a break from her son, she asked her husband to take over. "I get out of the house and head to Mecca Mall, buy a coffee and a croissant from Café Paul, and sit and watch the people go by. To clear my head, I mean. All mothers need alone time," she insisted. "And this is a problem with Arab women! They don't take care of themselves!" Umm Adil laughed appreciatively but countered Umm Fadi's suggestion. "I have my children to take care of! Plus, my husband would never accept this." Umm Fadi responded in an admonishing tone. "You must marry someone who has confidence in you! There must be confidence and trust!" Umm Adil objected to the implications of this reproach. "There is [trust]! But his mentality is simply different," she shrugged. "He didn't even want Lamia to attend university because it is co-ed!"

The conversation's easy transition—and gendered inflections—between child development, marital relations, and self-care offers one example of how discourses about modern womanhood and good motherhood contributed to making Down syndrome, as well as the class politics obfuscated by talk about "Arab women." Umm Fadi's advice relied on comfortable access to capital. Mecca Mall, while not the most elite or securitized mall in Amman, is nevertheless located in the upscale northwestern neighborhood of Khalda. And the current cost of a coffee and croissant at the café serving as Umm Fadi's refuge is seven dinar (approximately ten U.S. dollars). Then there is the question of free time and the related concept of "me time," neither of which resonated with Umm Adil. I did not know Umm Adil as well as I did Umm Fadi, but her black abaya and veil, juxtaposed against Umm Fadi's penchant for slacks and sweaters, suggested that they occupied different socioeconomic positions despite crossing paths through the shared experience of mothering a child with Down syndrome.

The interaction reminded me of a similar exchange I observed while attending a workshop for mothers of adult children with intellectual disabilities at a nongovernmental organization in East Amman. The guest speaker's white capri pants and bright-blue blouse set a stark contrast against the women sitting in front of her, most of whom wore jilbabs and hijabs in black or muted colors. Engaged in a more general conversation about including children in household routines and responsibilities to cultivate a sense of purpose, she urged her audience to establish boundaries and make sure their children understood that mothers need time for themselves (she did not, however, suggest including spouses in this messaging). Most of the women in the audience met this counsel with blank stares or cynical smiles. After a moment of quiet, an attendee finally replied with "Sa'ab" (It's difficult), wearing a polite but wry expression on her face. The speaker was sympathetic but unconvinced. "No one will give me my rights if I don't take them," she offered as a didactic rebuttal.

While Umm Fadi emphasized trust between spouses and the speaker promoted self-care and boundaries, fear also emerged as an important site of intervention.[15] In both its excess and absence, fear proved problematic. To fear for someone (*bikhaf 'alayy*) was to love them. Yet too much fear could become an impediment or even harmful. Where should one draw the line? In an early intervention session with the toddler Lujayn and her mother, Batool sought to ascertain whether Umm Lujayn had been practicing the drills and activities assigned during their previous appointment. As she proceeded through her checklist, Batool expanded her questions to inquire more generally about Lujayn's daily activities and routine. Umm Lujayn began to blush, her youthful face framed by her black hijab and white underscarf. She occasionally shot nervous glances in my direction while responding mostly in the negative to Batool's questions.

BATOOL: Do you let her play on the swings?
UMM LUJAYN: I'm afraid [Ana khaifeh]!
BATOOL: Have you considered enrolling Lujayn in swim lessons? Swimming is very good for the muscles.
UMM LUJAYN: I'm afraid [Ana khaifeh]!
BATOOL: Umm Lujayn! Strengthen your heart [Bit'awi 'albek]. Children learn from each other. Lujayn is lonely.

Batool turned back to Lujayn and began testing the next skills on her agenda. Umm Lujayn's fear became a problem, from Batool's perspective, when it created obstacles to the activities and experiences that would facilitate Lujayn's development. Quietly, however, and speaking more to herself than to anyone else, Umm Lujayn responded to Batool's rebuke. "She's not lonely. Wherever she is, I am." Focused more on the vertical tie of their mother-daughter bond than Lujayn's lateral ties to other children, Umm Lujayn understood her fear as a healthy expression of love; no one would fear for her daughter like she did. Other mothers articulated similar sentiments, expressing intense anxiety about letting their children with Down syndrome socialize with peers, let alone cultivate friendships outside a close circle of siblings, cousins, and neighbors whose families they knew well.

In a session with Umm Leen and her baby, Leen, Batool suggested that the child seemed excessively unsettled by her surroundings. Just prior, Batool had gently shaken a long purple sash with jingly bells tied to the end of it, sending Leen into fits of screaming and tears. Umm Leen looked thoughtfully at her infant daughter, wrapped in a bright-pink snowsuit and bearing a striking resemblance to an oblong fluffy marshmallow. With a pensive but deliberate tone, she replied, "It's better [that] she fears than not fear." Umm Leen saw Leen's fear as an appropriate tool for navigating a hostile world, enabling her to remain alert to its dangers and complexities. Batool worried about Leen's fear becoming debilitating. This (potential) impairment acquired its own sociology in the context of Jordanian motherhood and womanhood (Hughes and Paterson 1997).

Differing degrees of fear shaped how women perceived each other, evaluated their children, and assessed their broader environments. Even if early intervention could ameliorate or prevent developmental delays, how would this translate into a broader social milieu that they considered profoundly devoid of acceptance? One morning I attended a gathering at Al-Nur that Umm Farha described to me as a mothers' support meeting. The attendance, however, proved lackluster. Umm Adil arrived first, without Adil, and Umm Farha asked why she had not brought her son. Somewhat surprised by the question, Umm Adil explained that she saw the meeting as a rare opportunity for rest. "If I brought him, he would be holding my hand the whole time. . . ." She trailed off and focused on drinking the cup of coffee that Umm Farha had given her in welcome. After Umm Adil, a young woman named Suha entered the building. Because she felt like a second mother to her younger brother with Down syndrome, she hoped that attending the meeting would be informative and helpful for her whole family.

We settled into the plastic chairs while cupping our hands around requisite paper cups of instant coffee. Umm Farha asked the group, "What's the hardest thing facing our children?" Umm Adil responded immediately: "Society [al-mujtama']. I'm afraid people will laugh at him, exploit him." Umm Farha pushed back. "These fears are appropriate to every child. Why do we think they're unique to children with Down syndrome?" Suha chimed in. "We have to fear for them a little more." And Umm Adil added, "I'm afraid of him being out and alone." Umm Tasnim, who joined the conversation after finishing her early intervention session with Tasnim, reinforced Umm Adil's and Suha's arguments. "Tasnim can't talk," she offered. "I'm afraid of losing her, and she won't know how to get back or to ask someone for help." Umm Farha, however, did not waver in her position. "These are *our* fears, not theirs."

In their back-and-forth, the group disagreed about how to intervene and on whose behalf. Umm Adil and Umm Tasnim described their children as uniquely vulnerable, with Umm Adil emphasizing the cruelty of society and Umm Tasnim emphasizing the risks heightened by her daughter's limited speech. Umm

Farha did not refute their concerns about society or its exploitative and often cruel nature. Nor did she minimize the challenges of raising a mostly nonspeaking child. But she criticized Umm Adil for exceptionalizing Down syndrome, and she urged Umm Tasnim to disentangle her own fear from what Tasnim might fear—and desire—for herself. Through these negotiations, Umm Farha worked to shift the gaze of intervention from children's bodyminds to family members and the obstacles they created when they centered their own beliefs and emotions. Ultimately, a host of actors participated in mapping the habilitative terrain of early childhood with Down syndrome, including children, mothers, husbands, sisters, teachers, and peers (which is to say nothing of nonhuman actors: bouncy balls, markers, clay, books, Google). For most of my interlocutors, God also participated in these habilitative encounters, shifting questions of scale and design beyond those detailed in any Portage guidebook.

INTERWORLDLY INTERVENTION

Whether speaking with a special educator employed by a charitable organization, a mother who volunteered to organize awareness campaigns on social media, or a human rights activist well versed in disability legislation and the United Nations Convention on the Persons with Disabilities, most women navigated the ambivalent interventions they faced and followed with an understanding that disability comes from God.[16] This situated disability as a site of "interworldly" (Friedner 2019, 2020) intervention that invited women to work on their relationship with God and their faith by embracing and advocating for their child.

Umm Iyad first learned of her youngest son's Down syndrome over a month after his birth, when she returned to the doctor for her own postpartum checkup. Mentioning Iyad's low birth weight, the doctor informed her of his suspicions. When I asked about her initial reaction to Iyad's potential diagnosis, she hesitated briefly and her voice dropped. "It was difficult . . . difficult. There was no awareness. I didn't know anything Down. No one even called it that. Even the doctor said 'mongholi.' Yet the very first thing I did was say alhamdulillah, alhamdulillah, alhamdulillah" (all praise/thanks belongs to God). In that moment, she was grateful for her close relationship with God and her relationship with her husband.

Despite an overwhelming and almost unbearable sense of shock, she went to the hospital mosque and prayed. The waiting period between the doctor's informal assessment and the official diagnosis was the most challenging part. The doctor said he was 90 percent certain that Iyad had Down syndrome, but what about that other 10? Before and after a chromosomal test confirmed Iyad's Down syndrome, Umm Iyad used *du'a* (individualized supplication) and *salat* (ritualized prayer) to sustain herself. She told me: "I didn't depend on other people to lighten my burden. I worked on myself. I have conviction [*qana'a*]. If someone has any problem or disaster, if they are not from their heart accepting and convicted . . . Alhamdulillah this is something from God. Everyone talks, but I have conviction. I worked on myself—du'a, salat, closeness to God. I became closer to God. I felt that was a test and a lesson for me. I became closer to God, alhamdulillah." Gradually, the shock dissipated, and she and her husband turned their attention toward explaining Down syndrome to Iyad's siblings and then more gradually to their larger family network.

Umm Iyad's interworldly intervention set the terms for her initial encounter with Down syndrome and the choices she subsequently made for herself and her family. She continued working (rather than leaving her job, an outcome she initially anticipated would be inevitable). She became an active member in volunteer and outreach opportunities. And she prayed, which she described as work on herself. Acceptance required a relationship with God, and that relationship required self-work through prayer. While some self-identified "religious" women interpreted an absence of acceptance as symptomatic of moral failure (see chapter 2), Umm Iyad approached acceptance as a process. In doing so she extended the parameters of acceptance beyond herself or her son as individuals, and even beyond their mother-child partnership. Umm Iyad cultivated her relationship with her son in and through her relationship with God, and vice versa.

When I met Umm May and her family, first introduced in chapter 3, they were living in one of eastern Amman's most neglected neighborhoods. First-, second-, and third-generation Palestinian families have historically called Jabal Ahmar home, but Iraqi and Syrian refugees have also resettled to this less prohibitively expensive part of the city. While Umm May prepared the family lunch, her sister-in-law, Alia, suggested that we pass the time and entertain May by taking a walk. She wanted her own chance to respond more privately to the questions I had posed about shock and disability, and she wanted to introduce me to her neighbor and friend Umm Samira. We strolled through Jabal Ahmar's narrow alleyways, where undulating rows of cement buildings were stacked closely together on winding inclines and valleys. This made strolling a concerted effort even during the limited stretches of temperate weather.

Taking time to catch our breath, Alia narrated a unique oral map of her adopted neighborhood by pointing out various households and naming disabilities experienced by the residents inside (Down syndrome, blindness, deafness, cerebral palsy, intellectual disability). Rather than "hidden" or "taboo," these various domestic states of well-being and divergent embodiment formed an unremarkable—or, at the very least, unavoidable—part of the community's social fabric. When we arrived at Umm Samira's home, our host appeared confused by my presence, but she graciously invited us inside. Alia explained that I was visiting their family to learn more about May and more about how Muslims understood disability.

While my interlocutors overwhelmingly identified as Muslim, Alia herself introduced this qualification to her friend. I never explicitly mentioned religion when describing my research to participants or interested parties, instead using the more general category of "culture" (*thaqafa*). Although most of my interlocutors regarded religion and culture as analytically distinct, their practical entanglements proved important to answering the questions I asked and to navigating their everyday lives. Umm Samira responded to Alia's introduction by showering me with several *masha'allahs* (literally, "God wills it," a phrase of appreciation and acknowledgment) and *habibtis* (my dear), inviting me to join the Qur'an study group that she and Alia attended. She then went to bring Samira into the room.

Samira was the youngest of Umm Samira's six children and her only daughter.[17] Physically and intellectually disabled, Samira experienced extensive brain damage after birth as the result of what Umm Samira described as *dumur al-'aql* (cerebral atrophy), a category used to describe a variety of cognitive disabilities.[18] Neither verbal nor ambulatory, Samira watched and engaged the world around her from a bodymind whose size and communicative capacity remained significantly constrained. Umm Samira bluntly listed her daughter's extensive impairments by providing a litany of diagnostic labels and ailments. She also made a point to mention that whenever one of her brothers approached her—they often assumed responsibility for feeding their sister—Samira would break out in laughter as a way of saying hello and thank you.

Alia explained that I had asked about her family's shock on learning of May's Down syndrome. She stressed the word "shock" and paused, giving her friend a knowing glance, and then added, "Christine has heard that people here interpret disability as a punishment from God." The comment caught me off guard because I had never mentioned this claim to Alia. It did, however, surface throughout my fieldwork, most frequently among activists and foreigners working in Jordan's humanitarian and development sectors, or among elite Jordanians who sought to distinguish themselves from the masses. This detail perturbed Umm Samira, and she immediately responded to counter any misunderstanding on my part. "Habibti! How could Samira be a punishment? She is my path to heaven. She is proof that God loves me. She is mine and of me. How could I reject her?"

The idea that a disabled child creates a path to heaven, and I use the word "child" here to signify a kin relationship rather than a particular age range, emerged at various points during my research. While "of" their parents, to quote Umm Samira, children ultimately came from God. Caring for a disabled child increased the merit or reward (*'ajr*) that accompanies the good deed of care (Jansen 2004).[19] All children are blessings from God, and caring for any child increases one's 'ajr. But many family members and disability professionals interpreted intellectual disability as erasing the "account" by which adults are judged. According to the Qur'an, those for whom "the pen does not record against" are guaranteed a spot in heaven, which intensifies the stakes of their relationships with others (Ghaly 2019).[20] This model does not fit with a humanitarian or even a humanist framework of care. Instead it points to an interworldly moral rubric (see chapter 3) guiding how some of my interlocutors made and made sense of Down syndrome.[21] The value accrued through this nonaccountability, however, also came with costs that I will return to in chapter 6.

Alia turned to me, wanting to clarify further: "Umm Samira accepts her daughter's disability." Then she paused and thought about it. "No, she submits. This is the meaning of Islam, to submit. This is more than acceptance." At that point Samira became agitated, and Umm Samira briefly retreated into their home's interior to find Samira a snack while we remained in the salon designated for receiving guests. "Without faith, you cannot accept this," Alia said, her eyes not leaving Samira. "[Without faith] you cannot survive." In seeking to explain Umm Samira's experience, Alia drew on a relational repertoire exceeding that of acceptance. She reframed her neighbor's relationship to disability as one of submission. Acceptance did not contradict submission, but the latter surpassed the secular boundaries of the former. When we returned to Alia's family home for lunch, Umm May wanted to know where we had been and who we had seen. Alia told her about our visit to Umm Samira, describing Umm Samira's hospitality and Samira's general status. The family viewed Umm Samira's situation as particularly difficult because Samira was her only daughter. While reflecting on Alia's report, Umm May reminded us that Samira's impairments had no bearing on the wholeness of her soul (*ruh*), a critical interworldly component of her disabled bodymind.

INTERVENTIONS AND TRANSITIONS

Portage reformatted early childhood with Down syndrome through assessment meetings, checklists, and abstract standards of being "on track." As evidenced by Umm Shuruq, most women welcomed this intervention, even as they found paradoxes of bodily plasticity challenging to navigate. Did acceptance entail an uncompromising pursuit of developmental benchmarks, or did it require a radical rethinking of "normal" timelines and measurements? Could they find some form of compromise between these two poles? Would they know how hard to push and when to stop? Beyond embodied immediacies and uncertainties of developing Down syndrome bodyminds, the spaces, practices, and policies that coalesced during early childhood generated new ways for women to relate to their children, to themselves, and to each other.

The first time I met Umm Farha, she told me about the trauma of receiving Farha's diagnosis. The doctors doubted that Farha would survive infancy, and she experienced heart complications that required immediate surgery. During their early years together, Umm Farha experienced overwhelming anxiety, wondering what kind of child Farha would become (a very funny and very stubborn child, as it turned out). I asked why she decided to fight the grim prognostications of her doctors and the uncertainty conveyed by her family and friends. What led her to accept Farha's Down syndrome so unequivocally and convinced her to reorganize her own life and become a vocal advocate? She responded without hesitation and quite matter-of-factly, as though the question was straightforward and perhaps even simple. "I believed in the rights of my child. God gives us chances. Why would I take them away from her?"

Umm Farha's response did not minimize her own dedication to Farha, but she anchored this commitment in her relationship with God. If she did not advocate for her daughter, she would be depriving Farha of something that was not hers to take—God-given chances. Yet Umm Farha did not minimize the labor that intervention demanded. "I love Farha. My role as a mother is to try and help her to the best of her ability. But I'm exhausted. The challenges will never end." She did not anticipate an easier future. Farha would always have Down syndrome, and they would continue to face the challenges of living in a society (and world) that did not truly accept disability. That is why she relentlessly pursued advocacy work that nevertheless took an obvious toll on her—with fatigue, headaches, anemia, and dizziness.

The future was unlikely to get easier, but she could work to make it better. This meant pursuing interventions that would help Farha develop to the best of her ability while also cultivating relations of responsibility across their family, especially between Farha's siblings. At that point, Farha remained squarely within the realm of childhood. Unlike the many parents who equivocated on the importance of inclusive education, Umm Farha spent much of her time fighting to make sure that Farha could access public schooling alongside her nondisabled peers. But aging beyond childhood, which I turn to in chapters 5 and 6, invited new questions about bodymind capacity and the gendered modalities of making Down syndrome.

5 · GETTING STUCK

"Lucky you!"

"Christine!" Nahida called out. I spotted her face in the crowd, her eyebrow arched in disapproval at my late arrival to the Ramadan iftar. The gathering was sponsored by a youth group that invited Al-Nur Society and other disability-focused initiatives to break their fast while enjoying music, dancing, and face painting. These acts of volunteerism intensify during the month of Ramadan, which can make for a very busy social calendar. "Did you come here alone?" Nahida asked me, equal parts intrigued and aghast. "Where is your family?!" I chuckled at her bewilderment and reminded her that my family were all in the United States. So, yes, I had come alone. She then leaned in and whispered conspiratorially, "Lucky you" (Niyyalik)!

The recurring health problems that Nahida faced as part of her life with Down syndrome made her physically vulnerable to illness, but they did not diminish her sass. Nahida's mother also faced chronic health issues, which had transformed into periods of acute crisis on more than one occasion. Nevertheless, she maintained a close watch on her beloved daughter despite the latter's stated desire for more space. Both women enjoyed recognition for their active social life and commitment to public outreach efforts focused on changing perceptions of Down syndrome. Occasionally, however, they were the subject of gossip, with Nahida's form-fitting shirts provoking whispers. The resultant disapproval, however, fell equally or more so onto Umm Nahida as the presumed arbiter of Nahida's wardrobe choices.

To be clear, there is no consensus in Jordan about what dressing appropriately (or well) entails. Islamic notions of modesty inflect sartorial norms, especially in public spaces and events, but women incorporate religious identity, class, ethnicity, and individual preference into their personal style (Abbas 2015; Kaya 2010; Tobin 2016). In Nahida's case, however, reactions to her outfits did not reflect disagreement among members of her or her mother's social network, which consisted primarily of veiled women who wore *jilbabs* (a trench coat–like outer layer often belted at the waist) and "Western" outfits they modified to meet expectations of coverage. Instead, they highlighted uncertainties about how Nahida fit into established categories of girl and woman, child and adult.

Scrutiny over Nahida's wardrobe brings me back to the mothers and special educators who urged me to concentrate my research on aging and Down syndrome. In doing so, they contrasted dilemmas of growing older—which they situated as a familial process—against the unproblematic or relatively less problematic years of childhood. Even parents of younger children, who acknowledged the benefits of Jordan's ongoing expansion of disability advocacy and services, expressed acute anxieties about aging and the passing of time. Their worries often coalesced around puberty (*al-bulugh*) and adolescence (*al-murahaqa*).[1] The more medicalized connotations of these terms distinguished them from that of "youth" (*shabab*),[2] which holds political significance across Southwest Asian and North African (SWANA) countries.[3]

With burgeoning exposure to popular health and psychology media, and especially through social media, parents associated adolescence with hormones and unrest (both physical and emotional).[4] Puberty prompts observable changes in how adolescents dress, interact with their elders, and engage with peers, especially those of the opposite sex (Kaya 2010; Meneley 1996). Many experience this phase as "betwixt and between" (Turner 1967), or a "liminal state" between childhood and adulthood (Turner 1969). Yet for young women and men with Down syndrome—and for anthropologists skeptical that *etapes de vie* (van Gennep 1961) accurately capture the social process of aging—adolescence engendered more intransigent contradictions of change and stasis.

VITAL CONJUNCTURES AND EMBODIED ASYNCHRONY

The "problems" introduced by aging with Down syndrome and the "solutions" that some families pursued stemmed from a perceived misalignment between young people's embodied capacities and social proficiencies. This misalignment, or *embodied asynchrony* (Kafer 2013, 48), funneled young people into "stuckness" between roles and life stages (Sargent 2021).[5] While often treated as self-evident, life stages actually take shape as the cumulative effect of social projects. "When lives are not built in the interstices of formal institutions," notes the cultural demographer Jennifer Johnson-Hanks, "'entry into adulthood' loses even this apparent coherence" (865).

For young people with Down syndrome, who were often excluded from formal institutions like school, work, and marriage (a point I explore more fully in chapter 6), puberty engendered what Johnson-Hanks describes as "vital conjunctures." Resisting the fixity ad boundedness implied by a "life stage," vital conjunctures encompass "a socially structured zone of possibility that emerges around specific periods of potential transformation in a life or lives" (Johnson-Hanks 2002, 871). Significant moments and experiences—such as dropping out of school (Esson 2013), parental death (Evans 2014), or pregnancies foregone and lost (Hall 2022)—can all precipitate vital conjunctures. For adolescents with Down syndrome, the intersection of puberty with intellectual disability became a vital conjuncture, generating "experiential knots during which potential futures [came] under debate and up for grabs" (Johnson-Hanks 2002, 871).

Neither inevitable nor inherent to adolescence with intellectual disability, embodied asynchrony congealed as families aged and struggled with daily and sometimes exigent pressures of providing and receiving care. Amid these struggles, mothers prioritized an ethos of protection over one of autonomy. Most understood themselves as custodians of their children's bodily and reproductive futures, even as they imagined those futures on wide-ranging and sometimes conflicting terms. The strategies that some parents employed to manage—or attempt to resolve—embodied asynchrony included sterilization and behavior-altering medication, while others deployed less invasive but no less impactful methods of surveillance and immobilization. None of these practices are unique to disability in Jordan (Block 2000, 2007; Vaidya 2023), but Jordanian social, religious, and legal institutions created distinct conditions for navigating them. These practices also generated widespread debate and dissensus, which I address later in this chapter.

As a key institution for molding the arc of kinship futures, marriage anchored local constructions of embodied asynchrony. Jordanian legal and medical institutions reinforce a widely held norm that sex should only occur only between spouses. This expectation informs social scripts—and fears—around puberty, sexuality, and growing older (a point that connects this chapter with the next). Children born out of wedlock in Jordan lack "lawful lineage" (*nasab*) and are legally considered orphans, a designation that engenders stigmatizing and discriminatory consequences (Engelke 2019; Farahat and Cheney 2015; ICKHF 2017). Reproductive health is subsumed under the mantle of "family planning" and remains a sensitive topic even among married women (Alyahya et al. 2019). Parents are reticent to discuss puberty and especially sex with their children (Almasarweh 2003), while school-based sexual and reproductive health education receives little investment from the state despite documented parental support for expanded programming (Gausman et al. 2019; Othman et al. 2020, 2022).

Intersections of age, gender, and sexuality set the terms for embodied asynchrony and shaped the limits of what could be asked and said and how. Discussions about daughters and puberty tended to be quite clinical, with menstruation made discursively manageable by disconnecting it from related topics of sexuality and desire. Discussions about sons included frank references to masturbation, but they possessed a similar clinical directness. The unevenness of these conversational parameters reflected a broader sensibility that discussions about sex are most appropriate between spouses. This informed how women broached these topics with a foreign ethnographer, especially one who was neither a wife nor a mother. Mindful of these considerations, not to mention my own culturally informed sensitivities, I welcomed the information my interlocutors offered but less proactively pursued follow-up questions.

Ultimately, embodied asynchrony did not emerge from within the boundaries of individualized bodyminds. Instead, it materialized through the relations of care and harm that structure horizons of imagined—and feared—kinship futures. In much of this chapter, I explore how families of young women with Down syndrome (and other intellectual disabilities) navigated embodied asynchrony by drawing on the social, legal, religious, and medical institutions that organize vital conjunctures of Jordanian adolescence. I then turn to the intersections of gender and intellectual disability that led young men, much like their female counterparts, to also become increasingly stuck between the possibilities of childhood and adulthood.

ENACTING EMBODIED ASYNCHRONY

I first met Mona while observing a workshop on inclusive education. When I explained my research interests to the program attendees, all of whom were studying special education at the bachelor's or master's level in universities across Amman, Mona urged me to speak with her mother. "I have two sisters with intellectual disabilities," she exclaimed, keen to make the connection obvious. A few months after the program concluded, we reconnected via WhatsApp, and Mona invited me to visit her family in their home, located on the edges of eastern Amman. As the small bus (known as a coaster) progressed toward the Zarqa governorate, I noted the shifting aesthetics. The white limestone of Amman's western and central neighborhoods faded into yellowing stucco facades. A graffitied figure of Handala—the outline of a ten-year-old child turned away from viewers, his hands clasped behind his back—stood out among other symbols of Palestinian solidarity, which were spray painted onto cracked and crumbling cement walls.[6]

Already waiting for me as I disembarked, Mona and her mother waved me over to their car, which was piled full of goods from a recently concluded shopping trip. I squeezed into the back seat, and we took a short drive to their family home, where they ushered me into the salon reserved for guests. Lina, one of Mona's three sisters, stood waiting for us. Earlier that day, I had left my glasses in a taxi, so I sheepishly resigned myself to wearing my (prescription) sunglasses in the dimly lit room while apologizing for the awkward fashion statement. Being extremely nearsighted, I cannot bear even a few blurry hours of going without my visual aids. Whether to ease my embarrassment, or perhaps because she liked my style, Lina ran to get her own sunglasses, the kind with plastic neon frames that come in shades of blue, green, and pink. She donned them in solidarity, and we sat together in our shared semidarkness.

Mona then went to bring her youngest sister, Hala, into the room, while their other sister Nur also joined us. A wheelchair user, Hala was neither speaking nor ambulatory, and her extremely small body size reflected the presence of a global developmental delay. Umm Lina then sat down with her four daughters and, after the obligatory proffering of coffee and snacks, began to tell me about their family. Unlike some parents, Umm Lina offered a decidedly optimistic outlook on disability rights and culture in Jordan. She embraced an imaginary that contrasts Jordan's modern, progressive present against a grim past, and she did not lament the current moment as one of unrealized potential or disappointment.

Touching on questions of acceptance, shame, and hiding—with the importance of marriage cutting across all three—she explained that "there's more acceptance now. A long time ago, people would hide them [people with disabilities] and stay in denial and not speak about them. And maybe, in cases of marriage, when people would come to ask for a girl's hand, her father and her grandmother—the father's mother—would tell her not to say anything. Even my own mother . . . would ask, 'Does everyone who enters your house have to see [Hala]?' And I would tell her that Hala is part of our life, and people need to know that she is present." Echoing narratives explored in chapter 3, where solidarities between lineal and affinal kin differentially shaped the aftershocks of diagnosis, Umm Lina identified husbands and their mothers as primary sources of conflict but then adjusted that model. Even her own mother attributed a sense of threat to Hala's disability, fearing it would become a liability to her sisters' marriages.

Lina's impairments were not as readily apparent as Hala's. Then in her late teens, she moved independently and possessed a far greater capacity for speech than her younger sister. Yet Lina, not Hala, garnered more intense concern from her family. At different points throughout her life, Lina received diagnoses of developmental delay (ta'akhur namawwi), intellectual disability (i'aqa 'aqliyya/ dhihniyya), and a psychological condition that her mother described as akin to schizophrenia (zayy al-infisam). Mental illness compounded her intellectual impairment, creating what her mother described as "severe" (shadid) disability.[7] Umm Lina did not consider Lina's childhood easy, but the onset of puberty precipitated intense conflict inside their family and beyond it. While Umm Lina's narrative was challenging for me to follow, she made herself crystal clear on one key point: She considered the onset of Lina's period a disaster.[8]

Bodily fluids are intimate, sticky, and pungent substances that can quickly become disruptive as "matter out of place" (Douglas [1996] 2002). Having to manage them through collaboration can challenge deeply felt boundaries of privacy and intimacy. The symbolic and practical aspects of menstruation create additional considerations for observant Muslims completing wudu', a state of physical and spiritual purity that must be met before every prayer. Umm Lina, however, emphasized that *Lina* found her periods unbearably painful and could not understand what was happening to her body, let alone adequately manage the necessary hygiene practices. So Umm Lina began seeking information about preventing or stopping her period. This is when she crossed paths with rights activists working to assess the extent of hysterectomies performed on women and girls with disabilities.

Jordan does not share the legacies of state-driven medicalization, institutionalization, and sterilization that inform most Western (and some Eastern) disability rights movements. But many disabled people in Jordan, like their counterparts around the world, are still denied access to sexual and reproductive health services and prevented from creating the families they desire.[9] Given Jordan's relative absence of state-driven eugenics, I understand family-driven quests to manage sexuality and reproduction as forms of "everyday biopolitics" (Fullwiley 2004). Debates around hysterectomy (*izalat/isti'sal al-raham*; literally, removal of the uterus), irrespective of how commonly it occurs, reflect a contemporary iteration of long-standing communal and legal anxieties around the sexual and reproductive lives of persons deemed "not normal" (Moghnieh 2022; Scalenghe 2014).

Umm Lina did not specify how she first encountered the activists, but she vividly recalled their arguments. She began by affirming her respect for their work but expressed confusion over the boundaries they drew between care and harm. In recounting their conversation, Umm Lina was struck by the argument that a hysterectomy would violate Lina's right to motherhood (*haqq al-umuma*). To this, she responded: "Lina is fundamentally a child! In the center, they request that we delay the age at marriage and do not marry girls too young.[10] Then they go back, even with this mentality, and say that it is a girl's right to be a mother. But [Lina] is a child, and she will stay a child for her whole life. They are not very logical!" Umm Lina pitted the liberal discourse of children's rights against the ethos of bodily autonomy and reproductive freedom nurtured by disability rights movements.[11] Efforts to eliminate the marriage of minors— particularly girls—exist across Southwest Asia and North Africa and receive considerable funding from local, regional, and global initiatives (Sweis 2012). By locating Lina in perpetual childhood, a category accompanied by an unassailable right to protection, Umm Lina sought to physically align her daughter's body with this designation.

The obvious paternalism of describing adolescents or adults with intellectual disabilities as children clashes with the political and ethical sensibilities of global disability rights politics. Outright dismissal of this rhetorical strategy may miss its importance in sustaining "a disability appearance" not otherwise possible (Zoanni 2019, 448). Appealing to "childhood" can affirm personhood when its basic recognition comes otherwise under total threat. Analogies between intellectual impairment and childhood in Jordan also reflect the influence of Islamic scholarly and legal traditions that utilize this strategy (Ghaly 2019). The experiences of young women like Lina, however, highlight the gendered costs of such an appearance. Childhood may facilitate access to personhood, but the resulting embodied asynchrony becomes grounds for violent forms of bodily intervention, such as a medically unnecessary hysterectomy.

Kinship futures, as a Jordanian lens of "time and futurity" (Kafer 2013, 20), structured the intersections of gender, disability, and sexuality. Many women in Jordan never marry, but the prematurely determined impossibility of Lina's marital and maternal future, given her status as a disabled and "lifelong child," made her body especially problematic for those around her. As a family-planning method, sterilization appears to be uncommon and unpopular in Jordan. So do injectables and implants (Khalaf et al. 2008). Of the 60 percent of currently married women using contraception in 2023, most relied on withdrawal or intrauterine devices (20% each), followed by the pill (8%) and the male condom (6%) (DOS and ICF 2023, 111). Only 2 percent of currently married women were sterilized, and fewer than 1 percent used injections or implants (DOS and ICF 2023, 112).[12]

Importantly, providers and patients understand these methods as tools for *family planning*. When women like Umm Lina sought medical advice for their daughters, they turned to professionals for whom marital futures circumscribed possibilities for sex and desire; the absence of an imaginable marital future placed both outside the limits of discourse and practice (a point I return to below). With cessation of menstruation as the stated priority, methods of intervention that controlled fertility without stopping periods (like tubal ligation) would not meet their goals. While alternatives to hysterectomy that reduce or stop periods without having an impact on fertility do exist, parents and advocates used the terms *izalat/isti'sal al-raham*. It is possible, however, that some used these phrases as a general label for distinct methods of period control, not all of which entailed sterilization (*ta'qeem*).

More immediately than through encounters with biomedicine, embodied asynchrony materialized through relations with kin. This is where multigenerational social networks grappled with the dilemmas engendered by practices and conflicts of care. "Lina's sisters are at the age when they should be getting married. Should I prevent them from getting married [to take care of her]?" Umm Lina asked, repeating for me the question she had posed to the rights activists who challenged her interest in pursuing a hysterectomy for Lina. They refused to entertain this line of reasoning and affirmed that Umm Lina's other daughters most certainly could and should get married. This brought Umm Lina to what she considered the crux of the issue. "Okay. But if I die and her sisters get married, or if I get sick, who will change her? Her brother?! Her father?!" She offered the latter options for dramatic flair and to highlight their wild inappropriateness. Ultimately, Umm Lina's mother worried about a future in which she could not care for Lina—or for Hala. Hala's relatively "unproblematic" status reflected an unequal sense of "urgency" engendered by each daughter. As the youngest daughter, and the one who more easily and visibly fit into the category of "child," Hala remained profoundly dependent on others to meet her basic survival needs. Lina was not visibly disabled, which intensified her family's fears around her vulnerability to exploitation or manipulation.

Umm Lina anticipated her own eventual absence from her daughters' lives and recognized that she might become unable to serve as a primary caregiver well before that point arrived. She hoped that Mona and Nur would eventually share responsibility for their sisters. The alternatives—a limited number of state-run institutions or wildly unaffordable private centers—were largely unthinkable. Care, as a precarious resource that remains overly dependent on the availability of women kin, inscribed gender and disability onto Lina's body and into her relations with others. They converged to make embodied asynchrony a reality through the prism and limitations of kinship futures. And yet, as neither biology nor destiny, embodied asynchrony materialized through intersubjective relations. As a result, not all families experienced puberty as a traumatic rupture.

CONTESTING EMBODIED ASYNCHRONY

Reflecting on her daughter Rana's menarche, Umm Rana explained quite matter-of-factly that "it was fine. Alhamdulillah it just went smoothly. [Rana] learned how to take care of it and take care of herself. It was normal." Umm Rana did not frame menstruation as innately problematic, nor did she relegate her daughter to a state of perpetual childhood; instead, she located Rana squarely within the realm of adolescence. But this evaluation hinged on Rana's capacity for self-care as "normal." If Rana could not "take care of herself" and instead required the assistance of others, would her mother have resorted to more extreme measures? Umm Rana acknowledged that some families pursued hysterectomies for their daughters, and she made no explicit judgment on this choice. She nevertheless described Rana as a typical teenager, just one who happened to have Down syndrome. And while she felt conflicted about her teenage longings, she considered them completely reasonable *for someone her age.*

When I visited their home in an upscale neighborhood in northwest Amman, Umm Rana began to talk more about the paradoxes of aging. She told me:

> I don't like how [people] joke with them, like they don't take them seriously. . . . A while ago—she (Rana) loves watching Turkish soap operas, you know, and some of them are very open. She turned to her father and asked him, "When will I be able to fall in love? When I'm eighteen?" Can you imagine!? Dear God, ask me that, not your father! But she really means it! At least she was asking first [she laughed and shook her head at Rana's considerateness]. . . . But they are really

thinking about this stuff. They want this. Don't treat them like children because they don't see themselves that way.

This was not the first time we had discussed the uncertainties of adolescence. Months earlier, Umm Rana told me about a conversation she had with Rana that left her unsettled.

> Rana told me, "When I get married, I want to have six kids." I told her, "Six?! Who's going to take care of those?!" We have a maid, so she told me "Don't worry, I will bring two maids!" I told her, "You should take care of yourself first!" They're normal feelings for people their age. Of course, when her friends are getting engaged, she's going to say, "When is it my turn?" But my view is that at the end, it will be me, my husband, and Rana. In the end, we will be three.

Umm Rana objected to the infantilization that Rana and her peers experienced when nondisabled people diminished or even belittled their stated wants and needs. Yet she could not bring herself to envision the future that Rana imagined for herself.

Rana's parents considered her uniquely vulnerable to abuse and exploitation, a preoccupation shared by many parents and one I return to later in this chapter. Sitting in the kitchen while Umm Rana prepared lunch and Rana watched an episode of one of her beloved Turkish serials in the next room, Umm Rana explained that the proximity of programming factored crucially into Rana's options as she aged out of school-based options. Beyond availability (cost was not a primary concern, making their family a notable exception), Rana's parents opposed any commitment in which Rana "could end up the first or last one on a bus." She meant this quite literally. The impact of transportation logistics on daily life made Umm Rana even less able to conceptualize a future in which marriage served as Rana's entry point into adulthood. Hovering on the edge of a different dilemma than Lina, Rana nevertheless found herself similarly negotiating the grip of embodied asynchrony.

In contrast to Umm Lina and Umm Rana, Umm Maryam's plans for her youngest daughter, Maryam, refused embodied asynchrony. Yet the relationships Umm Maryam hoped to facilitate for Maryam still depended on gendered entanglements of disability and care. Sitting with Amina, her eldest daughter, Umm Maryam made it clear that she fully supported the right of people with Down syndrome to marry, but with certain qualifications. "I hope I can marry Maryam to someone *without* Down syndrome, so he can take care of her. A woman with Down syndrome can give birth to a healthy baby, and then that baby can take care of her later in life."[13] This kinship future conformed to normative, traditional gender roles—Maryam as wife and mother. Yet it also portended a radically more independent existence for both mother and daughter. Umm

Maryam did not configure this vital conjuncture by thinking of either Maryam or herself as autonomous individuals. She imagined Maryam's future as interwoven with her own, and the future she desired informed the life she strove to build for Maryam. If Maryam married and became a mother, Umm Maryam anticipated that her own care obligations would lessen in her older age.

When we broached the subject of hysterectomy, I anticipated Umm Maryam's response, given her hopes for Maryam's marital and maternal future. Yet in explaining her stance on the issue, Umm Maryam concentrated less on what a hysterectomy would mean for Maryam's potential motherhood than on the question of its religious permissibility. "Hysterectomy is haram, forbidden in Islam! God made her with a uterus! [Allah khala'ha ma'a al-raham]. Who am I to take that from her?" Her words echoed those of Umm Farha, who reasoned at the end of chapter 4 that because God gave her daughter chances, she was obligated to fight for those chances. Both women articulated an ethos of accountability that grounded care between kin in a broader Islamic cosmology. Umm Maryam recalled her disbelief when she learned that some women were willing to consider hysterectomies. "Mothers say they're afraid of their [disabled] daughter getting pregnant. Why would she be in a position where she'd be capable of getting pregnant? Do you let her wander the streets?!"

She extended this argument to nondisabled women to demonstrate the fallacy of its reasoning. "People fear their daughters—healthy daughters—having relationships and getting pregnant. But do they talk about taking out their wombs?!" Umm Maryam was not trying to trivialize the seriousness of an illicit relationship. At one point during our conversation, Amina asked me if it were true that girls in America could go out as they pleased. She expressed jealous approval when I granted that unmarried American women might (though not always) experienced more autonomy in their daily movements than many of their Jordanian peers. As Amina listed off her highly structured daily routine to not so subtly demonstrate that she lacked the opportunity to "go wherever she wanted," Umm Maryam protested the implicit criticism. "I fear for you," she exclaimed. "*I have to.*" She turned first to Amina, then to me, and exasperatedly threw her hands up in the air when we declined to validate her argument. Umm Maryam did not deem either of her daughters as less deserving of protection. She treated them as valuable and thus also vulnerable in their gendered identities, which she sought to preserve by protecting their marital futures.

PROTECTION AND PERSONHOOD

Umm Maryam's objection to the legitimacy of hysterectomy hinged on gendered dimensions of kinship futures and God's role in shaping those futures. Because human bodies "belong to God," extraction or alteration can amount to an ethical violation, as evidenced by scholarship on organ donation in Muslim-majority countries like Egypt and Turkey (Hamdy 2012; Sanal 2011). These same concerns appear in religious scholarship on hysterectomy. In 2014 Jordan's Department of Ifta' (Fatwa Department) issued a formal decision on the question of sterilizing women and girls with intellectual disabilities.[14] Fatwas are not legally binding in Jordan, but as a recognized source of moral authority, their decisions are meant to inform the spirit of the law.[15]

After collecting testimony from medical, child development, and human rights experts, gathered at the behest of disability advocates, the council ruled *against* the permissibility of hysterectomy on the basis of intellectual disability. Its reasoning, which can be accessed via its website, outlines an ethic of bodily integrity that foregrounds God's sovereignty over all bodies rather than a liberal commitment to an inviolably sovereign subject-in-body. Decision No. 194, 2/2014, "Forbidding hysterectomies of girls with disabilities and society's obligations toward them" (Hurmat izalat arham al-fatayat dhuwwat al i'aqa wa masu'liyya al-mujtama'a tijahun), states that

> it is not permissible to undertake the removal of a [body] part made by God except in cases of illness that can be cured by this procedure. As for those with an intellectual disability or illness, we do not see this type of operation as permissible, as it infringes on God's creation, poses health risks through the surgery, and has the negative effect of enabling abuse and causing harm and damage to these girls. It is the duty of parents and guardians to protect their daughters with intellectual disabilities and to spare them what may harm them, just as it is society's duty to offer them protection from exploitation and enact the necessary [legislative] measures to ensure this. It is the right of the weak to their protection. (Dar Al-Ifta' 2014)

The text articulates four interrelated objections to hysterectomy: (1) It infringes on God's creation, (2) the risks of the surgery outweigh the benefits, (3) it has the negative effect of enabling abuse and causing harm and damage, and (4) it denies women and girls with intellectual disabilities their right to protection.

Umm Lina, Umm Rana, and Umm Maryam shared a commitment to this ethos of protection and the imperative to mitigate harm. Their divergent perspectives on the "scale and scope of the problem" nevertheless influenced their respective stances (Hamdy 2012, 170). Umm Lina sought to protect Lina—and the rest of the family—from an embodied asynchrony that reached beyond the boundaries of Lina's bodymind into her relationships with those around her. "Who will care for her?" she asked repeatedly. The scholars who drafted the fatwa positioned women and girls with intellectual disabilities as subjects for whom care is a human and a God-given right, defining care first and foremost in terms of protection. In their formulation, the capacity for pregnancy preserves the body's ability to testify if that protection fails. In other words, eliminating the potential for pregnancy (through sterilization) eliminates an obvious indicator of sexual misconduct or rape. The department was not indifferent to the challenges of providing care. Responding to an earlier online query from the mother of a thirteen-year-old seeking an opinion on hysterectomy, the council similarly denied the operation's permissibility (Dar Al-Ifta' 2009) but urged the petitioner to locate the appropriate social services to support them. Ultimately, however, it prioritized the ramifications of altering the body in ways that would remove its capacity to reveal wrongdoing.

The disability rights activists who challenged Umm Lina presented a similar argument, that sterilization can lead to concealed sexual abuse, but their delivery refracted Jordanian politics of religion and class. Umm Lina conveyed visible rage when recalling their argument that pursuing a hysterectomy for Lina amounted to protecting her daughter's (potential) abusers (which implied that her husband or one of her sons would be the most likely perpetrator). Elsewhere, I also encountered this discourse among Jordanian elites, who described sexual abuse as endemic among poorer people because of their "traditional" collective sleeping arrangements, as well as a more general diagnosis that religiosity and poverty lead to sexual deviance. The coloniality of this narrative—which does not diminish the seriousness of the issue—offers another example of how Jordanian imaginaries interpolate disability through a well-worn vocabulary of backwardness, tradition, and violence. What these different logics and arguments share, however, is their understanding of pregnancy as a form of testimony.

Legal mechanisms have since emerged to reinforce the fatwa's nonbinding opinion. The Law on the Rights of Persons with Disabilities (Law No. 20 of 2017) contains several articles that undermine the legality of sterilization. Articles 5 and 30, respectively, affirm the necessity of obtaining informed consent for all medical procedures and the right to bodily integrity. Law No. 25 of 2018 on Medical and Health Liability explicitly states that performing a hysterectomy without the written consent of the patient and approval from a medical committee amounts to a criminal offense and will result in hard labor and fines. Ostensibly, the procedure could also fall under the jurisdiction of Article 335 of the Criminal Code, which addresses unlawful cutting, amputation, or disablement. Amendments to the Criminal Code initiated by the Higher Council for the Rights of Persons with Disabilities (HCD) have also intensified punishments for all crimes committed against disabled persons. Their 2017 Response to the United Nations Convention on the Persons with Disabilities (CRPD) oversight committee nevertheless acknowledged that medical professionals were under-educated about disability rights principles or the social model of disability, which contributed to persistent gaps between law and practice.

Pluralistic legal and ethical landscapes are not limited to Jordan; reports in Palestine and Syria describe similar instances of families "shopping around" to find doctors willing to perform a hysterectomy (El-Mohammad 2019; Jabril

2021). More recent media coverage in Jordan still relies on older data, typically citing the 2012 CRPD *Shadow Report* that placed the number of hysterectomies performed on girls and women with disabilities in the previous year at sixty-four cases (Alazzeh and Civil Society Coalition 2012, 121). The author, Dr. Muhannad Alazzeh, expressed doubts about the accuracy of that figure since the procedure can be justified as medically necessary to treat other health issues, like tumors and fibroids (Alazzeh and Civil Society Coalition 2012, 122).[16] In replying to the "List of Issues in Relation to the Initial Report of Jordan" in 2017, Jordan's response team stated that zero hysterectomies had been performed at public or private hospitals since 2015.[17] While they interpreted this as a sign of the fatwa's success, it is also possible that operations have moved further underground or into the less-regulated private sector. This very concern can be gleaned from a 2023 campaign convened by disability and women's rights organizations under the banner of "For Them," which sought to address continued familial and medical support for the procedure (SIGI 2023).[18]

Before these newer legal frameworks presumably shifted the willingness to go on record, some doctors appeared quite comfortable expressing a prosterilization stance. In a BBC Arabic article (Shadid 2009), two doctors employed by the Islamic Hospital (a private hospital established in the 1980s) and Al Bashir Hospital (the oldest and largest public hospital in Amman) described the sterilization of girls and women with disabilities as "a mercy for their families." An *Amman Net* article from this time quotes a gynecologist at Al Bashir who "defended the compassion of the operation and argued that 'the girl is not fit to become a mother, and she will not marry. . . . The family fears that there will be problems with her, like she will be raped and have a disabled child, and how could she care for him?'" (2007). While acknowledging the possibility of rape, this doctor appeared more concerned by the scenario of a disabled rape survivor giving birth to a (disabled) child.

When I mentioned this to Reem, my friend with a master's degree in special education from a private Islamic university, she shook her head in frustration. "Hysterectomy is forbidden in Islam. People with some disabilities, like Down syndrome, they can get married! Plus, it's not about rape, these arguments, they just fear [she made the gesture of a pregnant belly with her hands]. And then there's a baby with no father and a mother who can't take care of it." Conversations about sex between unmarried individuals occurred in the context of broader concern about children born out of wedlock—whether as the result of consensual or nonconsensual sex—who become the responsibility of maternal kin and cannot legally claim the right to patrilineal belonging. The dangers an unmarried pregnant woman might face from her own family further compounded this concern. And while Reem acknowledged that people with Down syndrome could marry, the dominant framework for these debates assumed the future unmarried status of the girl or woman in question.

Islamic, legal, and biomedical institutions created different conditions for constructing—and contesting—embodied asynchrony. The medical professionals quoted above marked the boundaries of women's bodies through technologies of surveillance and deindividualized relations between kin. They treated hysterectomy as neither solely nor even primarily a benefit (or a risk) to the woman in question but rather as a "mercy" for her family. The burden of care, from a biomedical perspective, made embodied asynchrony into a problem that surgical or chemical realignment could resolve. (Increasingly, however, activists and journalists are enlisting biomedical knowledge and authority to instead highlight the many negative side effects of early or unnecessary hysterectomy.) Umm Maryam and the fatwa, by contrast, located bodily integrity within individualized boundaries that could not be compromised for the concerns of kin. The latter stance did not align with the values of bodily and sexual autonomy that inform a liberal disability rights perspective, but it nevertheless facilitated their arrival at a similar conclusion.

Debates around hysterectomy revealed widespread fears about intellectually disabled girls and women being exploited by their own families and by other actors and institutions tasked with providing care. These fears are evident in the position crafted by the Council of Ifta', which describes hysterectomy as potentially "enabling abuse," as well as by families and activists who condemned the practice on similar terms. In this framing, reproductive capacities become a kind of "truth-telling" mechanism able to hold carers accountable, while the question of disabled women's own wants and desires remain secondary at best. While assumptions about men's sexuality failed to surface explicitly, they nevertheless formed an implicit part of these arguments.

GENDERING EMBODIED ASYNCHRONY

Young men also confronted embodied asynchrony. Deemed similarly vulnerable to exploitation and abuse, they experienced tactics of heightened surveillance and protection, but many also enjoyed a greater degree of privacy and freedom. This gendered interplay of autonomy and constraint became especially clear when speaking with mothers of older sons. Young women's desires were cloaked in euphemisms of finding a boyfriend or husband, while menstruation appeared as a medical challenge.[19] Yet with a degree of frankness that chafed against my own culturally constructed inhibitions, I found myself listening to women the same age as my mother (or older) discussing the logistics of male masturbation.

While by no means a universal attitude, the matter-of-factness with which some older women segued into the topic conveyed a sense of banality, bolstered by a broader recognition of men's sexuality as public knowledge. In other words, men's desires—and evidence of those desires—were not considered as private or taboo as women's. Many women drew on medical or biological discourses to frame male masturbation as natural, albeit something warranting strict regulation; a dissenting minority insisted it was haram (religiously forbidden). These dynamics became clear while visiting a support group hosted by an organization located in a poorer neighborhood of East Amman.

The organization had invited a professor of special education to talk with mothers about puberty, and one woman took the opportunity to ask how she could prevent her son from masturbating. The speaker launched smoothly into a defense of masturbation as completely natural and probably practiced by all young men. (Based on the quizzical expressions of the attendees, I am not sure this resonated with everyone.) As mothers, the professor continued, they had a responsibility to teach their sons where they could engage in this practice and what to do afterward, especially with regard to properly washing one's body and dealing with soiled clothes. She also suggested that if it rose to the level of a problem, she would first ask herself, "Why does he have all this free time in his room alone?!" While neither unnatural nor completely reprehensible, such expressions of desire needed to be controlled.

My conversation with Umm Ali revealed how patriarchally gendered logics created conditions for enabling or resisting embodied asynchrony. When Ali was young, his mother had advocated for him at a time when medical and educational services were not readily available, and Jordan's disability rights movement had only begun to gain momentum. With Ali now grown and in his late twenties, questions about aging, meaning, and purpose preoccupied both mother and son. Before turning to the topic of marriage, Umm Ali spent some time opining on the complications of puberty. In doing so she reversed the explanation endorsed by Umm Maryam and the Council of Ifta'. She considered hysterectomy more than reasonable for young women with Down syndrome, and she stressed its purported religious legitimacy.

> I support it, and so does Islam. If my daughter had Down syndrome, I would have to remove her uterus. It's better for her, and it's better for her mother. If she got her period, it would be such a challenge. Let her be comfortable. And girls have sexual desires more than boys; that has been proven, scientifically. With a boy, you need to look out for him twenty-four hours a day, so imagine how much harder is it to look after a girl? You need to be even more on guard.

The same argument, however, did not apply to boys:

> When there is a boy, I am against the idea of a mother going to a doctor for medicine to lower his sexual desires. Because it of course affects him. . . . So, it's wrong that the mother of a son who has Down syndrome then causes him to suffer from another condition. It is wrong that a mother with a boy with Down syndrome should have to have even more problems. It is his right to live his life.

Hysterectomy, according to Umm Ali, benefited both mother and daughter (by removing the stress and pain of menstruation). Administering libido-reducing medicine, however, could have a negative impact on the health of a boy or son (she switched between these terms but did not use the word for man, *rajil*).[20] Consequently, she could not condone it. (This is part of why activists are now trying to marshal biomedical knowledge to communicate the health risks of unnecessary hysterectomy.)

In this utilitarian framework, when a marital future was deemed impossible, menstruation became an embodied and disposable nuisance, nature made strange through circumstance. Young men, however, presented a different set of considerations. "A boy grows up," Umm Ali told me. "I mean, it is no problem, teach him to go to the bathroom. That's his right to get his sexual desires out of his body. Watch out for him. Teach him to go into the bathroom, to wash and clean himself; this is normal. But he cannot do it in front of people!" Describing masturbation as easily contained and managed by the individual, Umm Ali's stance reflected broader assumptions about gendered bodies, sexuality, and subjectivity. Discussions about sons registered self- and other-oriented heteronormative desire, but discussions of daughters only recognized other-oriented expressions of heteronormative desire and with far less detail. The vulnerability that parents imputed to disability and the sexuality generally associated with adolescence shaped making Down syndrome at this vital conjuncture, but gender by no means lent itself to uniform experience.

Umm Ayman lived in an affluent suburb of West Amman with her husband and Ayman, the youngest of her three children. Like Umm Lina, Umm Ayman described the onset of puberty as a dramatic rupture. When Ayman was young, everything was "normal," but things changed when he turned fifteen. Umm Ayman prefaced her story by remarking that it was difficult to talk frankly about the body and sexuality in the Arab world (*al-'alim al-'arabi*). "It's not that it's forbidden. There's starting to be more discussion. But the discussion is not honest, and it's not enough. And a mother, of a disabled son, can expect that at adolescence there will be hormonal changes." She followed this preface with a seemingly abrupt change of topic, recalling how, one day, Ayman refused to get off the bus during the morning drop-off at the expensive private center he had attended for years. Initially, I could not see how this moment connected to Umm Ayman's broader narrative, but I came to realize that the memory marked a turning point for her.

That morning struggle with the bus heralded behavioral and affective changes—anger, tics, and aggressive outbursts—that Umm Ayman connected to one main issue: "the bathroom." She then became more direct. "The masturbation influences his mind. We don't forbid him from entering the bathroom, but when he starts, our routine changes, and then there's conflict." The bathroom symbolized the disruptiveness of puberty and the frustrations of adolescence.

Ayman's family turned to medication to try to control his behavior, both "the bathroom" and the physical outbursts that were becoming increasingly common. The pharmaceuticals caused further problems. Ayman began having seizures, which his doctors then sought to control through more medication. This escalating cycle of drugs and side effects unfolded as Umm Ali outlined above, with medicines creating new problems and causing additional harm. Paradoxical stereotypes that paint intellectually disabled people as more aggressive and more vulnerable influenced how families protected—and policed—their children.[21] Mothers of sons, however, often identified women as the aggressors.

Umm Ali's daughter-in-law recalled an issue they had with a young woman with Down syndrome named Aziza who had tried to flirt with Ali. When she attempted to hold Ali's hand, Umm Ali recalled proudly, "Ali told her that this is not allowed. . . . 'Haram, haram!' I told him to hit her. He told me that he couldn't do that because it's not right." She chuckled at her son's level response and praised his maturity. "When Ali walks, he walks like this [she imitated someone with their arms tightly at their sides and their gaze lowered] and says excuse me so he can pass. His siblings take care of him and teach him." I smiled because this description captured my own interactions with Ali, who was indeed very cautious about maintaining embodied dispositions of propriety around members of the opposite sex.

Umm Ali's account reinforced popular depictions of female sexuality as dangerously powerful and of women as less capable of self-control (Abu-Lughod 1986; Mernissi 1975). While aggressiveness also plays a role in Jordanian constructions of masculinity, excessive roughness and violence are considered backward and un-Islamic (Hughes 2017). Aziza, who was close in age to Ali, occasionally voiced her desire to find a boyfriend. Yet she also actively participated in maintaining gendered moral codes of propriety. When attending events where music and dancing occurred, she refused to participate. I once saw her chastise her friend Lara, only a few years her junior, for shaking her hips in mixed company, a move she deemed too suggestive. Disability and sexuality shaped how both young men and young women like Ayman, Ali, and Aziza inhabited their gendered identities, which changed over time, but they all became increasingly stuck between childhood and adulthood.

ASYNCHRONY: EMBODIED AND EMPLACED

As teenagers like Nahida communicated their changing desires and attempted to enact new versions of themselves, their parents, siblings, and caregivers debated what was possible and what was right. I have followed how these deliberations played out among the latter by relying on partial stories told from mothers' perspectives, which are neither neutral nor generalizable. The chapter's narrative reinscribes the agency and authority of mothers (and parents) who wielded considerable power over their children. Their perspectives nevertheless provide insights into how inequalities of gender and generation intersected with disability to constrain the possibilities and choices that family members faced in striving to secure kinship futures.

Imagining the "life course" as a smooth progression between stages does not match how people experience aging and struggle to inhabit expectations of their socially constructed age. Yet embodied asynchrony attests to the symbolic and material power that this narrative still holds. Vital conjunctures emerge as individuals and families navigate extant expectations around gendered adulthood and shifting distributions of care labor. Because marriage is a key access point for socially and legally legitimate expressions of heteronormative sexuality, the perception—while changing—that people with Down syndrome could not or should not marry unsettled normatively cast kinship futures and intensified embodied asynchrony.

While situated in distinct political and moral traditions, Fatwa No. 194 of 2014 and Law No. 20 of 2017 on the Rights of Persons with Disabilities provided tools for resisting embodied asynchrony. They also provided mechanisms for facilitating the kinship futures that some young people sought for themselves. Nevertheless, children's potentially asynchronous misalignments between embodied and social performances of adulthood continued to preoccupy parents and other gatekeepers. They took divergent stances on how to navigate and reenvision the interdependencies that shaped and threatened kinship futures. Embodied asynchrony did not always precipitate overtly violent responses, like hysterectomy or forced medication, but more oblique tactics of control still precipitated frustration, unease, and confusion.

As a perpetual daughter in her parents' home, Nahida would remain under the scrutiny and care of her parents, and this arrangement would eventually transfer to her brother (and his hypothetical future wife). While Umm Nahida strove to provide her daughter with an active social life through educational and self-advocacy opportunities, those efforts took a toll, especially given her own unstable health. In chapter 6, I consider how embodied dimensions of aging intersected with spatial and material dimensions of house and home. These were the coordinates for crafting kinship futures and making Down syndrome as children grew up, families grew older, and economic and political conditions worsened across Jordan and the region.

6 · AGING UNCERTAINTIES

"As long as I'm alive…"

When I met Umm Fadi, her family was on the cusp of several life transitions. Her teenage son with Down syndrome, Fadi, was "aging out" of the educational and social programs available to him while struggling with his health, and their nuclear family was growing older. Umm Fadi and her husband had recently retired, while Fadi's older siblings had graduated from college and were starting out in their professional careers. As they embarked on these new life stages, their relationships and responsibilities toward each other weighed heavily on Umm Fadi's mind. Contemplating the future brought her to the topic of marriage, among others.

> I opened YouTube, and I saw that many families—even in Britain—have fears about the future of their children. . . . Some families have started accepting marriage. They marry their children with Down syndrome to each other. But even with marriage, [people with Down syndrome] need supervision from the mother and father. And their routine is a problem. . . . They don't remember their routine correctly, not on time. In Britain, they [people with Down syndrome] are educated and they can work, but they still need a mother or father supervising their routine. . . . So, mothers worry [there], and we mothers worry too.

Trailing off, she avoided making a final decision on the feasibility of this scenario, but marriage and its alternatives brought us to one of her core concerns about the future. "For me, as long as I'm alive, I will keep my son at home" (Badalni hafiz 'ala ibni fil bayt).

But what happens if Fadi outlives his parents? What happens if they can no longer support him in their own advancing age? How will they manage his changing needs alongside their own shifting capacities? Umm Fadi hoped that Fadi's siblings would commit to caring for their brother in one of their homes; that they would commit to keeping Fadi safe and healthy among kin. The only alternative would be to place him in residential care. Yet the Jordanian government plans to eliminate residential institutions over the next ten years, although they are already unpopular and relatively uncommon. Law No. 20 on the Rights of Persons with Disabilities asserts the right of persons with disabilities to live independently with their families or in community-based alternatives. But Umm Fadi did not want to assume that her other children would be willing or capable of taking on this commitment. Nor would she explicitly demand any such promise. It had to be "their choice," she explained, and only they could make it. She would leave things up to God and to time.

Umm Fadi's fears about aging point to the unsettled and unsettling questions that parents grappled with as they contemplated kinship futures in middle age and later life. These questions were not unique to families in Jordan, nor to families raising children with Down syndrome. But the convergence of disability and aging tend to intensify their gravity. In the United States, families describe this stage of life as akin to peering—or toppling—over a "disability cliff" (Ginsburg and Rapp 2024, 121; see also Bagenstos 2014; Bérubé 2018). The cliff forms as child- and adolescent-focused support services begin to dissipate, imperiling hard-won daily routines and narrowing life's possibilities. It is an ironic outcome of what anthropologist Pamela Block terms "unplanned survival" (2020, S70). While medical and social transformations allow more disabled and medically vulnerable children to survive into adulthood and beyond, the support systems required for them to thrive during the middle and later stages of life remain woefully inadequate. Beyond early childhood and removed from the urgency of serious illness or profound impairment are the relational dilemmas of parenting and disability "in the long run" (Whyte 2020; Block and Mcgrath 2019; Buchbinder 2015; Gammeltoft 2008, 2014a; Weiss 1994).[1]

This book offers a peculiar palimpsest of temporalities. My interlocutors talked primarily about memories or about experiences unfolding in a shared ethnographic present (that now also belongs to the past). This chapter focuses on futures that were then or are still yet to come. As parents grew older alongside children doing the same, relationalities of aging brought temporalities of care into sharp relief. Many mothers returned to shared preoccupations: Could and should their child marry? What would happen if they did not? Where would they go? Would siblings and their future spouses take them into their homes? What alternatives existed? How would they survive? How would they spend their days? And what would make those days meaningful? In grappling with these questions, parents repeatedly returned to practical and existential questions of home, marriage, and work, the building blocks of their kinship futures.

While separated for organizational clarity, these categories are interlinked and nondiscrete; each speaks to how questions of space intersect with those of time, age, gender, and embodiment. Contemplating aging and kinship futures generated acute anxiety, but it rarely elicited outward articulations of agony or dread.[2] Instead, families marshaled a diffident balance of humor, skepticism, and equanimity. Sobering geopolitical realities, historical and ongoing displacement crises, and faith in God tempered expressions of either despair or naive optimism. The future could be planned for, worked toward, and worried over, but it ultimately remained beyond the knowable—a point I return to at the chapter's close.

MOTHERHOOD AND DISABILITY "IN THE LONG RUN"

Umm Fadi highlighted education and work as compelling life pursuits, the first ostensibly leading to the second, whether alongside or in lieu of marriage. The limited feasibility of either, which she contrasted against their imagined accessibility in Britain, provided an unwelcome reminder of the many barriers that Fadi faced. These included economic precarity, high unemployment, and a growing emphasis on "knowledge economies." Yet in contemplating different possible futures, Umm Fadi remained skeptical that her British counterparts faced a reality so totally incommensurate with her own, despite what YouTube might want her to believe. She recognized a substrate of obvious worry as the connective thread between mothers "here" and "there."

The subtle and not-so-subtle reconfigurations of care that unfold through intergenerational transitions intensified familial concerns about building kinship futures alongside the realities of growing older. In theory, mothers of grown children had arrived at a point when their immediate care responsibilities would lessen. Their children and children's spouses would take on the labor of supporting new nuclear family units. Daughters and daughters-in-law would fund and source the elaborate dishes that drew families together for holidays and celebrations. Mothers of grown children could concentrate on delighting in the arrival of grandchildren who demanded less direct attention and investment. Rather than aging through the prism of a nuclear family, they expected to age in relation to connections and obligations between extended kin. Yet the increasing necessity of two-income households, a lack of affordable childcare, and chronically high rates of unemployment among traditionally male breadwinners have rendered this ideal somewhere between unlikely and unattainable.[3] The pressure to migrate west or east for better career opportunities has further fractured assumptions of lifelong intergenerational proximity. But even as shifting political economies of work and care continue to affect the actualities of aging, parents rarely cease parenting as children grow older. "Parent" is a relational status that does not so much wane as transform over time.

Many of the women I met spent their lives fighting battles alongside their children, whether they claimed the title of "activist" or not.[4] They fought for their children's right to access spaces not designed for them, to benefit from patchwork and unevenly available therapeutic and rehabilitation services, to enroll in school, to enjoy the extracurricular opportunities available to nondisabled peers, and to work in safe and dignified labor conditions. Expanding early intervention and educational programs infused earlier "life stages" with a sense of optimism, but the intertwined periods of adulthood (for children) and middle and older age (for parents) hastened new uncertainties and disappointments. Worries about *where* adult children with disabilities would live served as a medium for questions about *what* they would do, crossing paths with the equally compelling question of *who* could be counted on to ensure continuity of care and quality of life. These worries materialized in a social context where marital status, gender, and class viscerally regulate how bodies move through space and which spaces are deemed appropriate, safe, and desirable—or not—for differently gendered and aged bodies (Elyachar 2011; Ghannam 2011; Meneley 1996).

Conversations about "the future" often hinged on questions about marriage (even when mothers deemed marriage as practically out of the question), reflecting the role of marriage in constructing Jordanian adulthood. Yet disability also catalyzed critical reflections on whether marriage should or even could serve as such a powerful arbiter of adult status, a shift hastened by broader changes in Jordanian marital patterns and trends (Assaad et al. 2017; Gebel and Heyne 2016; Krafft and Assaad 2012; Salem 2012). As connective tissue between individuals, families, and generations, marriage organizes the "generative labor" of care across the life course (Buch 2018).[5] Over time and with age, women gain power and independence by performing generative labor, and they eventually gain power and independence *from* it. They anticipate these shifts on the assumption that the next generation of daughters and daughters-in-law will replace them. Middle- and upper-class families, moreover, can deal with unmet care needs by leveraging an international division of [generative] labor to hire migrant domestic workers (Parreñas 2012).[6] Yet even as the generative labor force becomes more internationalized (for those who can afford it), moral economies of care remain anchored in home and kin.

Aging with Down syndrome created conflicts between adult children and mothers, which many women found difficult to resolve or even fully acknowledge. Unequal interdependencies of gender and age intersected with classed sensibilities and economic constraints to shape how families—but especially mothers—approached the question of "What comes next for *us*?" The stakes of these questions reached beyond personal and familial scales. The "right to live independently" and "the right to home and family"—Articles 19 and 23 of the United Nations Convention on the Rights of Persons with Disabilities (CRPD)—are core principles of disability rights movements around the world. They materialize in Jordan through various provisions of Law No. 20, as well as awareness-raising campaigns, know-your-rights initiatives, reports from the Higher Council for the Rights of Persons with Disabilities (HCD), and regional and international conferences.[7]

The CRPD's universalizing human rights framework, however, does not resolve the complexities of local circumstances. Nor does it necessarily accommodate the ethical commitments and moral philosophies that people bring to bear on their own projects of living and aging well later in life. To draw out the "friction" (Tsing 2005) between this global disability narrative and its local reception, I begin the following sections by highlighting relevant articles of the CRPD, which I juxtapose against ethnographic data. I have chosen to do so precisely because many Jordanians take these global mechanisms and discourses very seriously; this is especially true for disability rights activists and policymakers. For families, however, the "right" path forward became less clear over time. Scripts that had previously offered hope and moral leverage began to veer out of alignment with the priorities—and risks—they deemed most important.

HOUSE AND HOME

(a) Persons with disabilities have the opportunity to choose their place of residence and where and with whom they live on an equal basis with others and are not obliged to live in a particular living arrangement;

(b) Persons with disabilities have access to a range of in-home, residential and other community support services, including personal assistance necessary to support living and inclusion in the community, and to prevent isolation or segregation from the community.

—Article 19 of the CRPD[8]

"As long as I'm alive," Umm Fadi asserted, "I will keep my son at home." When mothers explained their opposition to residential centers, they rarely focused on the principles of freedom and choice championed by lawmakers and activists.[9] Instead, they highlighted a more expansive and relational moral economy. In Jordanian Arabic, *al-bayt* can refer to a physical domestic structure, a neo- or patrilocal settlement, and a genealogically traced kinship grouping (such as the Hashemites).[10] The term also conveys the emotional and symbolic affordances of home and family. Al-bayt is the Jordanian locus for what anthropologists Joao Biehl and Federico Neiburg describe as house-ing, or the "sensorial process by which peoples and houses co-constitute one another" (2021, 541). House-ing recognizes houses and people as relational and dynamic and enmeshed in each other's co-construction.[11]

In Jordan, house-ing is embedded in relations between lineal and affinal kin. Men are far more likely to inherit family property or have access to the cash required to build or rent a home (Ababsa 2017; Hughes 2016). Following Sharia precedent, sisters receive a lesser share of inheritance than brothers, and in families without sons, some portion of inheritance passes to male uncles and cousins.[12] Only one in four women receive the full property inheritance they are entitled to by law, and many surrender this right under pressure from family members (Ababsa 2017).[13] Living alone is stigmatized and financially out of reach for most, while living with nonkin is also considered unusual. Most university students commute to campus, and although some schools offer housing, these residences are primary occupied by international students. "Dormitories" house women who migrate to Amman looking for work and lack local relatives, allowing them to protect their reputations and assuage family members' anxieties (Adely 2024). Muslims and Christians share reservations about living arrangements formed outside the boundaries of kinship and marriage, and Jordanians who migrate west often find themselves artfully obscuring the details of European and North American accommodations.

If Fadi did not stay in his parents' home, where would he go? People considered residential centers as a negation of house-ing, standing in opposition to home and the personhood nurtured within. Centers (colloquially used interchangeably with "institutions") epitomized the "hiding" that animates Jordan's disability imaginary (see chapters 2 and 3). In 2019, the HCD, in collaboration with the Ministry of Social Development, the Lumos Foundation, Humanity and Inclusion International/Jordan, and EU funding partners, released a ten-year strategy for deinstitutionalization, which is a legal obligation under Article 27 of Jordan's Law No. 20 (and corresponds to Article 19 of the CRPD). The plan demonstrates Jordan's attunement to the global deinstitutionalization movement, which seeks to confront the legacies and ongoing abuses that occur in institutional settings.[14]

While the mass institutionalization of people with disabilities continues to haunt the United States, Canada, and various parts of western and eastern Europe, Jordan does not share this living history. According to the HCD, as of 2019, thirty-four institutions (twenty-two of which are privately owned) housed a total of 1,471 persons with disabilities; 883 of the enrolled residents (or 60%) were non-Jordanians from neighboring countries (HCD 2019, 4). Given the 2015 census's estimated disability prevalence rate of 11.1 percent, approximately 1.1 million disabled people currently live in Jordan; this means that a relatively small percentage of disabled people in Jordan are institutionalized. Given the lower prevalence of residential institutions, people associated segregation and confinement with home and kin as much as they did with centers. Nevertheless, deinstitutionalization remains a priority for the Jordanian government, as it does for the global disability rights movement.

Implicitly, deinstitutionalization activists and families agree on the reciprocal links between disability rights, dignity, and "house-ing." They diverge, however, on the question of "home." Article 19 of the CRPD mentions the concept of home as a spatial designation, qualifying the location for service provision as "in-home."[15] Clause (a) asserts that "persons with disabilities have the opportunity to choose their *place of residence* and where and with whom they live on an equal basis with others and are not obliged to live in a particular living arrangement" (my emphasis). In the CRPD's moral topography, a "good" residence facilitates inclusion into "the community," but for many Jordanians, a "good" residence should also be a home. The latter is hard to separate from family. The boundaries between house, home, and community, furthermore, are not always so easy to parse.

I met Dima, an autistic woman in her early twenties, while attending a Ramadan iftar in the city of Madaba. My former landlord Hala, a disability advocate from the governorate of Madaba, invited me to attend the event. When I arrived, I found her exchanging greetings with an older man, whom I deduced to be Dima's father, standing beside his daughter and another woman. Nonspeaking, quite tall, and very thin, Dima clutched a plastic water bottle in her hands. As she wandered contentedly around the room, she took great pleasure in observing the flows of water and light. Dima's father departed while Dima's caregiver, Linda, took a seat at an empty table, looking bored and keeping one eye on Dima's peregrinations. I sat down with Linda and learned that she was from a village near Irbid (located north of Amman). After completing her bachelor's degree in special education, she started work at a private day center for autistic children in northern Amman. When they announced that a former client was looking for a full-time caregiver for his adult daughter, she jumped at the chance. It came with a significant raise that allowed her to make biweekly trips back to visit her family. During those trips, Dima's father stayed with Dima in the cottage where she lived, next to the family's main house.

Linda described Dima's father as a good man who loved his daughter. But when he remarried after his first wife's passing, Dima became an unwanted figure in the new marital home. She took care to tell me that Dima's father was "not ashamed of Dima, or anything like that. When they host gatherings in the family diwan [meeting hall], he lets her wander around and stay by his side. But I've never met the second wife." When I asked if Dima had friends, Linda gave me an incredulous look. "She knows [knew] her mother, her father, me, and the guard [haris]. That's it." Interdependencies of death, marriage, and care shaped Dima's lonely life, testifying to the danger of romanticizing home as a place where kin cultivate community. At the same time, "community" may not so readily materialize in spaces and networks removed from kin. "While disability rights activists imagine deinstitutionalization as a mechanism of liberation, in which inhumane institutions are replaced by a continuum of community-based supports," the reality has proven more complex (Buch 2018, 22). This is especially true as neoliberal economic policies and social imaginaries intensify the structures of gender and racial inequality that "home care" industries rely on (Ehrenreich and Hochschild 2004; Parreñas 2001). Community can become a source of suffering as well (Davis 2012), recapitulating the logics of segregation and incarceration associated with institutions (Ben-Moshe et al. 2014).

A focus on deinstitutionalization in the Global North obscures how Global South countries receive and implement this mandate through their own disability histories and house-ing infrastructures (Giacaman 2023).[16] Some families expressed curiosity about house-ing alternatives, such as those facilitated by L'arche, a global network of inclusive communities and projects founded by Jean Vanier in 1964.[17] Three L'arche communities currently operate in Southwest Asia and North Africa—one each in Palestine, Syria, and Egypt. Only the Syrian site offers the residential accommodations elsewhere explored by anthropologists working in the United Kingdom and Uganda (McKearney 2017, 2020, 2021; Zoanni 2019). In 2017, Jordan's CRPD response committee reported that "some tentative measures were taken to create inclusive community environments for persons with intellectual disabilities, but they did not last long because of the lack of a mature understanding of the concept which led to its rejection by local communities" (19).

When discussing residential possibilities for adult children, parents (and other kin) found the prospect of unrelated individuals living together concerning and incompatible with their own understandings of good house-ing. They did not always distinguish between "the center" as a space defined by institutional hierarchies and "the center" as a potentially inclusive and egalitarian environment (as in homes run by L'arche). Parents were especially uncomfortable with the prospect of unrelated individuals of the opposite sex co-residing in the same building. In contemplating alternatives to kin-based residential arrangements, they unanimously raised concerns about sexual abuse, as well as the possibility of consensual but nonmarital sexual relations. The nebulousness of "community" could not compete with the concreteness of kin, and the latter informed how parents contemplated the trustworthiness of future house-ing.

Umm Khalil, for example, echoed Umm Fadi when speaking about her son Khalil, then seventeen. A divorced mother of three, she expressed fierce opposition to residential centers of any kind or scale, deeming them acceptable for only the most extreme of cases, "where the mother and father have passed away, and the grandparents are not able to take care of the child." She was horrified when her own neighbors enrolled their daughter in one such center (she did not specify ta reason beyond describing the daughter as "disabled"). She wondered how they could justify this decision as Muslims. "I consider these children an *amana* [a trust from God]. . . . God chose us, and they are going to go to Paradise. God doesn't judge this child. . . . We have angels on the right and left [shoulders] . . . but no one records for them. I'm jealous of them!"

The belief that intellectual disability afforded a unique kind of personhood appeared throughout my research, with many parents describing their children as "a path to heaven" or a "gift from God." Umm Khalil drew on a widely shared belief that people with intellectual disabilities do not "keep accounts" (*ma yuhasibu*) with the two angels who record an individual's good and bad deeds from birth until death.[18] By not keeping accounts, they facilitate more expansive opportunities for people around them to practice and receive the divine rewards/merit (*'ajr*) that come from providing good care.[19] Many activists regarded these beliefs as obstacles to appropriate, modern understandings of disability and disabled personhood. In the words of one exasperated advocate, "We're all gifts from God! People with disabilities are *people with rights!*" Parents were careful to point out, however, that *all* children are considered a trust from God, and caring well for any child creates *'ajr*.[20] Neither absolute nor unconditional, this merit relied on the quality of the care provided and its goodness rooted in particularities of home. Yet even at home, embodied performances of modesty, intimacy, and respect influenced how men and women occupied the spaces most closely associated with giving and receiving care.

MARRIAGE

1. States Parties shall take effective and appropriate measures to eliminate discrimination against persons with disabilities in all matters relating to marriage, family, parenthood and relationships, on an equal basis with others, so as to ensure that:
   a) The right of all persons with disabilities who are of marriageable age to marry and to found a family on the basis of free and full consent of the intending spouses is recognized;
   b) The rights of persons with disabilities to decide freely and responsibly on the number and spacing of their children and to have access to age-appropriate information, reproductive and family planning education are recognized, and the means necessary to enable them to exercise these rights are provided.

—Article 23 of the CRPD[21]

In summer 2021, Ibrahim Rashdan appeared on my Facebook newsfeed through a widely shared episode of the DW (German public broadcasting) program *JaafarTalk*. Sporting a scruffy beard and greeting the camera with a smile, he introduces himself and says, "My name is Ibrahim, and it's my right to get married just like everyone else." The next shot shows Ibrahim sitting next to a young woman named Nour. Both are beaming, dressed in formal attire, as music plays in the background. The text on the screen describes this event, their wedding party, as a dream come true. The video then introduces Umm Ibrahim and the rest of the Rashdans: Ibrahim, his parents, and his four siblings sit in their salon, chatting and drinking Arabic coffee. The camera zooms in on Umm Ibrahim, who explains that Ibrahim's success comes from his self-confidence, which his parents cultivated by treating him "exactly like his siblings, exactly like everyone else."

This was not Ibrahim's first time enjoying social media fame. In March 2018 the web-based program *Jordan Today* (*al-Urdun al-Yowm*) hosted an episode in honor of World Down Syndrome Day that included an interview between host Diala Dabbas, Ibrahim, and his mother. In the video, Umm Ibrahim recalls how their encounters with ableist barriers galvanized the family to action. "Why does my brother go to school, study, and go to work, and I don't?" Ibrahim asked. Denied entry to public or private school, he instead attended a special education center. Given the circumstances, his mother explained, "Our home became his school." The family later decided to move to Amman from their home in Kerak so that Ibrahim could have a greater chance of securing meaningful work. By the time of the interview, Ibrahim was proudly employed by the Marriott hotel chain, an opportunity made possible with support from his family and an Amman-based organization working to create employment opportunities for intellectually disabled adults. Secure in his job, Ibrahim set his sights on the next logical milestone. He went to his parents and asked them for help finding a bride. The disapproval from their broader community shocked Ibrahim's parents. "How can someone with Down syndrome marry?" people asked, not bothering to conceal their incredulity. "But if you actually meet Ibrahim," his father argued, "he'll change your mind." Ibrahim was not the first of their children to marry, but the process unfolded differently for him. The court required both families to obtain medical reports confirming their capacity, which they found strange but agreed to procure.[22] With these reports in hand, they proceeded with the paperwork and, of course, with planning the party. The *JaafarTalk* segment concludes by informing viewers that Ibrahim and Nour live together in his family's home, and he still works at the Marriott. Next on his list of dreams is starting a family. Ibrahim's story attests to the collective work that marriage requires. This effort is not unique to marrying as a disabled person, as matchmaking often involves expansive networks of gendered and intergenerational labor (Hughes 2015, 2021). Disability amplifies the roles that class and wealth play in facilitating marital partnerships, as well as how collective and inegalitarian interests among family members shape individual marital futures.

A conversation with Umm and Abu Sami demonstrated how marriage operated as a mode of future-making. Sitting in the salon of their rented and threadbare apartment in a working-class area of Amman, I asked Sami's parents what came to mind when they thought about the future. Abu Sami asked Sami, the younger of their two sons and then in his early twenties, to return to drawing in his notebook, which he had been focused on before my arrival. Sami obliged, and his father then turned to me. "When you say, 'the future,' are you asking if he will one day get married?" Abu Sami wove marriage so tightly into the fabric of his imagined future that he practically defined each in terms of the other. But before I had a chance to clarify, he continued, provoking a spirited disagreement with his wife. Abu Sami hoped he could marry Sami to "a girl like him" (with Down syndrome) but noted that "others" told him it would be impossible. Umm Sami interjected with a resounding "No!" She strongly opposed the idea. Abu

Sami asked his wife why she would be against Sami marrying, and their back-and-forth proceeded as follows:

UMM SAMI: So that he will not have a child like himself. Who will take care of them? Am I right? I am [old], and I take care of him. If he gets married to another girl like him, there will be two people who need to be taken care of.

ABU SAMI: He doesn't have to have children. But just so that he can learn to be responsible and have a life. Like other countries, where they try to have them depend on themselves, and they have real work. When he sees his brother get married, he will ask, Why not him? And he will get sad, frustrated. When he watches TV and sees two people in love, he watches closely. He gets happy and laughs.

UMM SAMI: Yes, of course. He has emotions and feelings! Huwweh insan [He's human]!

ABU SAMI: I hope that he will get married, even if they don't do anything. Just so that they can be two people together, so that they will be a family.

Sami's parents envisioned the future through gendered and generational preoccupations with generative labor, and they negotiated their respective preoccupations through different marital configurations.

Abu Sami focused on the affective and emotional dimensions of marriage that could provide his son with meaningful companionship and a sense of purpose. His own gendered positionality informed his stance on whether (and why) marriage represented a possible future. He wanted his son to "have a life" and envisioned him doing so in terms of a social-sexual contract of adult manhood that relies on work and marriage. Men are expected to provide for their families economically and materially. In doing so, they can successfully perform their masculinity and visibly express love and care (Nasser El-Dine 2018). Failing as a provider can even prove grounds for divorce according to Islamic law (Mir-Hosseini 2000; Tucker 2010), and it is certainly a cause for disapproval and social censure. Abu Sami's appeals to their son's feelings and desires, however, did not sway his wife.

Umm Sami focused on the pragmatics of generative labor. Because patrilocality in Jordan is still relatively common, sons often live near their parents, if not in the same building, depending on their financial resources. Older women anticipate that daughters-in-law will provide companionship and valuable domestic labor, contributing to meals, keeping house, and managing family social affairs. Umm Sami wondered what a daughter-in-law with Down syndrome—let alone grandchildren—would mean for her. She first objected to the prospect of Sami having children (the normatively assumed outcome of all marriages) and then to his marrying at all. Her concerns about the labor of raising children exceeded her concerns about the work required to maintain a marriage. Abu Sami, in contrast, was willing to imagine a marriage that consisted of "two people together" and demurred on the question of children. Neither of Sami's parents denied his personhood or ignored his longing for companionship and love. They disagreed, however, on what Sami's adulthood might entail, negotiating its relationality in terms of marriage and reproduction. Gender was not the only factor shaping their perspectives. The family had fled Syria's civil war in 2012, and their hopes for the future bore the weight of their displacement. Aging as refugees was not something they ever imagined, but they endured, and they adapted.

Despite their considerably different life circumstances, Umm Sami's logic of refusal shared much in common with Umm Ali, a mother and grandmother comfortably ensconced in Jordan's upper middle class.[23] When I asked whether people with Down syndrome in Jordan could or should marry, Umm Ali responded somewhat exasperatedly: "If I wanted to marry [Ali], I would have to meet the girl's parents, and their financial situation would have to be very good. Because they [people with Down syndrome] have expenses for medicine and food. . . . I am not able to take care of another like my son; it would be impossible. But if her [financial] situation was very good, and they take him for a month, and then I take him for a month, then . . . maybe." Umm Ali described the prospect of caring for two adults with Down syndrome as impossible (*mustahil*), and she couched her objections in material and economic terms. Expenses for food and medicine, and the more implicit toll that generative labor takes on the body-mind, even when performed with love and commitment, shaped her sense of impossibility. As mothers of sons, Umm Ali and Umm Sami anticipated that their hypothetical daughters-in-law would likely live with them (as was the case for Ibrahim and Nour). Would their sons' wives' needs then become their responsibility? Would their wives' families contribute?

Umm Ali connected the domestic limits of generative labor to the larger political economy of caregiving in Jordan, objecting to a disability imaginary that seemingly ignored these constraints: "We don't need any problems. . . . I would consider it ignorance [*jahil*] for us to marry them. Why? Why is it so important? Leave him alone. Let him be. Once, when these doctors from Switzerland came, they told us to let them get married. 'It's his life,' they said. You all [Switzerland] provide them with everything, but here it isn't like that! Why would I marry him? To carry his burdens on top of my own ['Iba'u fowq 'iba'i]? Should I ask his siblings [to help]? If the government helped a little and gave him a salary, I would get him married. But to make the whole thing my burden? It's impossible." Disability and development experts often deployed accusations of ignorance to critique local practices of shaming or stigmatizing disability. Umm Ali inverted their equation by obliquely accusing the Swiss doctors—paradigms of progressive disability policy and national prosperity more broadly—of ignorance. The thoughtless promotion of marriage, irrespective of local context and the constraints faced by families in Jordan, marked *them* as backward.

From Umm Ali's perspective, arranging a marriage for Ali would risk invert-ing the "patriarchal bargain" that women negotiate—and reproduce—as they age (Kandiyoti 1988). This bargain offers them increasing authority and maneu-verability over time, especially through their relationships with daughters-in-law. The fact that this bargain may fail to deliver or become wholly untenable under deteriorating political and economic conditions has not dislodged its importance in organizing this gendered construction of the life course. Like Umm Fadi and Umm Sami, Umm Ali also wondered whether and how much she could lean on Ali's siblings to help facilitate their brother's different possible futures. Siblings play significant roles in each other's lives, albeit in ways shaped by gender, age status, and political context (Ghannam 2013; Jean-Klein 2000; Joseph 1993), but parents were cautious of taking sibling ties for granted. How-ever genuine and deep the love between them might be, the challenge of making ends meet rendered sibling support networks unstable.

Umm Sami and Umm Ali both characterized generative labor as burdensome, but they did not describe their children as burdens. They shared pleasure and pride in how they cared for their families, and they embraced the joys of being cared for in return. The physical and financial demands of care, however, and worrying about future care, remained undeniably stressful. Care can foster soli-darity, especially when imagined (and performed) as collective labor among "crip kin" (Kafer 2019). But in Jordan, the "care webs" (Piepzna-Samarasinha 2018) elsewhere enacted as lifelines for mutual aid and sustenance remain enmeshed in ties between lineal and affinal kin. These relations are shot through with patriarchal configurations of expectation and extraction, and they have been deepened by austerity and financial precarity. Together, these forces con-verge to make marriage a continued matter of collective interest and risk. All three women invested time, energy, and passion into advocating for their sons, but aging introduced painful uncertainties that placed them at odds with their children in new and uncomfortable ways.

One day, Ali returned home clearly smitten with a new acquaintance he met while volunteering at an event. He showed Umm Ali the girl's picture on Face-book. Umm Ali first responded by pretending not to understand her son's inter-est. Then she tried to redirect his focus: "He started to ask me my opinion of her. I looked at her and asked him, 'Who is that?' I understand what he wants, but I pretend that I don't understand. He told me, 'This one! I am asking you what you think of her.' I told him, 'I don't like her at all. She is very arrogant.' I told him that I didn't like her at all, and that she was not pretty. He disagreed. . . . I changed the subject so that he would forget and talk about something else. But there was a period when he would talk about it a lot." After one such con-versation, a visibly upset Ali asked his mother, "Am I sick? Is that why I can't get married?" Umm Ali told this story without meta-commentary, and I wondered about the thoughts and feelings she left unsaid. When Ali was younger, Umm

Ali had offered her sewing services in exchange for securing Ali's spot in school because the principal had refused to accept him. She developed his speech therapy regimen, given the absence of alternatives at that time. She immediately left the hospital after Ali's birth when she sensed that the doctors did not share her commitment to helping Ali survive and thrive. Their family worked together to ensure that he would. These shared achievements brought them to their current impasse.

With a cheerful disposition and healthy sense of irony, sharpened over her six-plus decades on this earth, Umm Ali talked about Ali with evident pride. But she was adamant that she could not support his desire to marry, and she had the power to refuse him. The responsibilities women typically shoulder for childcare, but especially when attempting to secure support for a disabled child (Landsman 2009; Rapp 1999), not only persisted but sometimes increased with age (Fietz 2020). The fear of institutionalization—or worse, ending up on "the street"—and the need to calibrate limited care resources across years and between bodies meant that futures remained shared by and tethered to families. Returning to Umm Fadi's point at the beginning of this chapter, even in Britain, where education and work appeared more readily accessible and people with Down syndrome seemed to marry without facing as many obstacles, parental investment facilitated access to these opportunities (Thomas 2021). For many families the collective labor required to maintain and secure kinship futures demanded communally enacted—and asymmetrically exacted—sacrifice.

WORK

1. States Parties recognize the right of persons with disabilities to work, on an equal basis with others; this includes the right to the opportunity to gain a living by work freely chosen or accepted in a labour market and work environment that is open, inclusive and accessible to persons with disabilities. States Parties shall safeguard and promote the realization of the right to work.

—Article 27 of the CRPD[24]

Like so many mothers, Umm Jamila constantly worried about what the future held for Jamila, the middle of her three children. While her older son and youngest daughter traveled abroad to complete their degrees, Jamila and her family struggled to build a fulfilling daily life for a young woman with Down syndrome in her early twenties. Jamila was vocally dissatisfied with her options, which consisted mainly of going to a special education center that organized activities for intellectually disabled people over eighteen; she refused to attend with increasing frequency. "She wants to go to university," Umm Jamila explained. "She wants to work like her sister and like her father and make money." Jamila watched her family members, but especially her sister and her mother, pursue educational and work opportunities; she wanted the same for herself. School and formal employment offer women relatively recently accessible and potentially transformative opportunities to build relationships and skills outside the home, but women carefully weigh these expanding options alongside enduring expectations of marriage and motherhood (Adely 2012; MacDougall 2021).

Umm Jamila did not want Jamila's world to shrink, and she found hope in the possibility of a meaningful job. The question of work, alongside and in relation to marriage, highlights how intersections of gender, disability, and age made Down syndrome on the cusp of an uncertain adulthood. Umm Jamila prioritized cultivating Jamila's sense of self-sufficiency, foregrounding the value of independence. In elaborating on what this entailed, she explained: "I wanted to make sure that she would never need to rely on her siblings. I'm not going to live forever. When I leave her with her sister or her brother, or with people, I wanted to make sure that she wouldn't be a burden. . . . Everyone has their own life to live and their own responsibilities to carry. I wanted to raise her to carry her responsibilities by herself." Rather than contrast independence with relationships, Umm Jamila configured independence as something that emerged through one's capacity to build relationships while maintaining boundaries. Many parents similarly affirmed the value of independence, and they strove to build "independent children." They gauged the relative presence or absence of independence through the capacity to exchange with, provide for, and not "burden" one's kin. Independence, however, contained contradictions.

On the one hand, Umm Jamila proudly affirmed Jamila's independence in her role as a daughter and sister. She did not, however, consider Jamila *independent enough* to become a wife or mother. That independence meant being able to "carry the responsibility of al-bayt—cleaning, cooking, another man, children . . ." She trailed off momentarily and then continued. "I'm older. I'm not young. I must think practically and logically about these things. She cannot do all that on her own." Umm Jamila foregrounded her own mortality in explaining her opposition to Jamila marrying. She would not "be around forever" to help Jamila navigate marriage—or motherhood. She might, however, consider such possibilities under a different economy of generative labor. "Maybe if there was a . . . village, let's say, under the supervision of the government, with specialists on call to provide care, that could work. But she cannot handle those responsibilities alone."

Jamila observed that people her age were starting to marry, and she wondered when it would be her turn. Echoing Umm Farid, Umm Jamila admitted that when her daughter asked about this milestone, she usually tried to change the subject, or she raised the minimum age at which marriage would be appropriate. "At this point, she thinks that when she turns thirty, she will get married. But when she turns thirty, I'll tell her that she will get married at thirty-five." Employing a different tactic, she also tried reminding Jamila how much she needed her.

Who could Umm Jamila rely on to care for her as she aged if Jamila left her to get married? (It is quite common for an unmarried adult daughter to live at home and assume the primary caregiver role for aging parents.) Work could provide Jamila a sense of purpose and means for (greater) independence, but her options were constrained by Jordanian paradoxes of gender, inequality, and opportunity (Adely 2012).

Concerns about respectability and fears of harassment—at and en route to work—play a role in how women choose to both enter and exit the workforce (Abu Moghli et al. 2018; Aloul et al. 2018). Jamila once received an offer to work in the kitchen of a nearby hotel, but her parents "had to reject it" because they did not know any of her potential coworkers. They could not predict who might be "coming and going" in a place like that. Jamila was attentive, responsible, loving, and she adored children; her mother felt she would be well suited to work as a helper or aide in a nursery. But Umm Jamila correctly anticipated that strangers' misperceptions about Jamila's skills and talents would harm her capacity to enter this otherwise helpfully feminized field. Women with Down syndrome (and other disabilities) faced a gendered double barrier in their efforts to build adult lives: doubts about their capacity to marry and doubts about their capacity to work left them with few options (Abu-Habib 1997). Yet parents of sons also expressed fears about their children's vulnerability to exploitation. Even with boys, according to Umm Jamila, one had to worry. "I know mothers who, yes they are confident in how they raised their own son, but they can't trust how other people raise *their* children."

Sami's parents confirmed these fears in strikingly similar terms. Sami had previously worked in a local fast-food restaurant, but his parents grew wary of how his fellow employees treated him. They recalled a growing sense of unease as they watched some of Sami's co-workers fail to respect his vulnerability to coercion. If someone told Sami to do something unscrupulous, his father explained, he might go along with them out of his desire to please. One of his co-workers once encouraged Sami to smoke a cigarette. While another co-worker eventually stopped him, they worried about Sami's ability to "say no," whether to the pervasive practice of smoking cigarettes or to more untoward requests.[25] Broadly speaking, Umm and Abu Sami worried about the relationships Sami might form at work. At one point Umm Sami added that "even if [Sami] was not disabled, we would have to worry about these things."[26] While not untrue and widely echoed by mothers of sons, the degree of worry and extent of the power that Sami's parents exerted over him exceeded what parents would consider appropriate for a young man in his early twenties *without* Down syndrome. Sami's parents thus vacillated between the "doubled discourses . . . of sameness and difference" that play an ambivalent role in making Down syndrome over time (Rapp 1999, 293).

"NO ONE KNOWS THE FUTURE"

In the throes of everyday life, contingencies of aging alternately faded into the background and surged to the surface. But across this ebb and flow, some inevitabilities remained crucial to making Down syndrome and contemplating the horizons of kinship futures. At one point my interlocutor Hana shared that her mother found thinking about the future especially distressing, and she worried most about Hana's younger brother with Down syndrome, Jamal. Much like Umm Fadi, Umm Jamal would ask Hana, the third of five children and her parents' only daughter, "If I die, and your father dies, what will happen to Jamal?" Sometimes, Hana responded by problematizing the question itself. "We don't know. Maybe I will die first!" In retelling this exchange, she reaffirmed the soundness of her argument and added somewhat ominously, "It's not always the older generation that dies first. . . . Of course, I fear the future; [I fear] for everything in my life. We can't think too much about the future because it makes life hard."

Moral and practical dimensions of care connected siblings through kinship futures, and those connections changed with time and loss. Hana was close with Jamal, and she anticipated continuing to care for him like "the second mother" she had become. But as a divorcée living in her parents' home, both she and Jamal would become more vulnerable when their parents passed. House-ing can manifest kinship's continuities, as well as its vulnerabilities and inequalities. These include the transfer of wealth between fathers and sons (often to the detriment of daughters), the provision of bridewealth and housing by grooms to their prospective wives, and the expectation that adult children reciprocate the care that aging parents once provided to them. These social and legal structures shape generational transitions in quite literally concrete terms, through the concrete "pressed into cinderblocks, and built into houses that can be occupied by families dreaming of stable sanctuaries where they may safely dwell and prosper" (Hughes 2016, 1083). In avoiding her mother's plea—a plea for her to promise that she would one day take over—Hana felt it unwise—and perhaps impossible— to trust the normative trajectories cast by kinship futures.

7 · ACCEPTANCE

"Maybe I'll die first!"

Hana's mother feared what would happen to Jamal, Hana's younger brother with Down syndrome, when she and her husband passed. But from Hana's perspective, Jamal was not the only person whose future warranted concern. "Maybe I'll die first!" she argued. "Of course, I fear the future. I fear for everything in my life. We can't think too much about the future because it makes life hard." Umm Jamal's anxiety and Hana's equivocation betrayed a hard truth that both women understood all too well: Futures cannot be taken for granted. In Jordan, where historic and ongoing waves of mass displacement visibly materialize in social suffering and precarity, there is no shortage of reminders that imagined futures can quickly disappear or be stolen.

Dealings between global superpowers and their regional allies have always proceeded with little regard for those who suffer their consequences most directly. Kin are critical to weathering these storms. This includes the intimate familiars who make life livable, whether by circulating small sums of money on an endless loop of borrow and return, by scouting out the cheapest best produce at the souq, or by vetting the reputation of a potential employer. It also extends to less familiars and unfamiliars: cousins living in Gulf countries who help cover tuition; siblings of siblings by marriage who have relocated to Canada and can support visa applications; communities that share surnames, ancestors, and histories of interconnection but find themselves divided by arbitrarily drawn colonial borders of unimaginable consequence. Ties of genealogy and geography (amenable as they can be to adaptation and improvisation) preserve these reservoirs of opportunity.

Solidarities among kin, alongside their manifest fragilities and disappointments, shaped banal and consequential aspects of everyday life in Jordan, and they amplified the risks of stigma that traveled through relational networks. Families navigated these contradictions of connectivity while making Down syndrome through practices of care. In doing so, they interacted with—and largely welcomed—an expanding grid of public and private services that aim to establish and manage "disability" as a biopolitical category. Yet this grid continues to struggle, as political and economic infrastructures imagined by "global" instruments like the United Nations Convention on the Rights of Persons with Disabilities collide with the implementation capacities of the Jordanian state, of municipal governments, and of local communities. Alongside these newer mechanisms, kinship remains an enduring disability infrastructure. Intersections of patriarchy and ableism link mothers and children together, but they precipitate divergent consequences over life course and historical time.

ACCEPTANCE: MAKING AND BEING

"Before, there were not so many people with Down syndrome. Because they all died! They didn't know then what they know now—about their nutritional needs and their heart problems. *There wasn't any care!*" Umm Ali was sitting behind the reception desk at the Al-Nur Society, speaking to no one in particular. The grandmotherly figure introduced across previous chapters often shared reflections on how much had changed since her youngest son, Ali, was born nearly thirty years ago. At that moment, the reception room was filled with a not uncommon hodgepodge of children, mothers, other relatives, visitors, and special educators (and one errant ethnographer). Various motivations brought them together. Some were accompanying children to appointments, others were volunteering to fulfill administrative duties, and still others were dropping by to check in while running neighborhood errands. Their lives as Down syndrome families, or their connections to those families, pulled them into the same orbit, albeit with varying degrees of interaction and intimacy.

Umm Ali linked her perception of Down syndrome's increasing presence to improvements in medical and scientific knowledge. Lamenting the past and celebrating the present, she recapitulated the developmentalist trajectory that I have described as a core component of Jordanian disability imaginaries. Grounded in changing empirical realities of disability that Umm Ali herself had witnessed firsthand, this narrative also weaponizes care through a culturalist lens that depicts Jordan and its peoples as perpetually "behind." Better (health) care has undeniably contributed to the increasing life expectancy and expanding possibilities seized by people with Down syndrome around the world.[1] Yet these developments exist alongside a decreasing presence of people with Down syndrome in places where high rates of prenatal testing are followed by high rates of pregnancy termination. This seemingly opposite phenomenon also reflects an outcome of expanding health care; the contradiction speaks to the multiplicities of making Down syndrome in the current moment.

To understand Umm Ali's narrative of Down syndrome's "before" and "now," I have turned to "domains of kinship and reproduction as key social sites at which [disabilities] are initially assigned cultural meaning" (Rapp and Ginsburg 2001, 536). But I have gone further by suggesting that kinship and reproduction are also key social sites for *making* Down syndrome through the prism of kinship futures. In dialogue with other disability futurities, like crip (Kafer 2013) and sensory (Friedner 2022b), I use kinship futures to highlight how the networks and temporalities of care that make Down syndrome in Jordan remain tethered to networks and temporalities of kinship. Far from static or unchanging, kinship futures adapt and respond to the historical and political circumstances that impinge on everyday life. But their horizons of possibility are enmeshed in ideologies and practicalities of kinning (Howell 2003, 2006).

The impacts of expanding knowledge and improving health care appeared in many of my interlocutors' stories, but they were never the whole story. For this I return to Abu Yehya and his description of acceptance as "the most important thing." Acceptance reappeared in various moments and encounters: processing the shock of diagnosis, training bodyminds through early intervention, grappling with the costs and benefits of educational arrangements, contemplating appropriate outfits and viable vocations. Through these dynamic negotiations, acceptance forged existential knots between the making of Down syndrome and kinship futures. In considering such knots, I draw on the anthropologist Michael Jackson's approach to *being* as "a perennial struggle for existence . . . a dynamic relationship between the human capacity for life, and the potentialities of any social environment for providing the wherewithal of life" (2005, xii). Acceptance created ways of being and being-with Down syndrome.

Some anthropologists remain wary of "being." João Biehl and Peter Locke lean on the philosopher Giles Deleuze (and Félix Guattari) to contrast being with becoming. They embrace the latter, arguing that becoming "destabilizes the primacy of *being and identity* in the Western philosophical tradition in favor of attending to shifting sets of relations and the ongoing production of difference in the world" (2017, 8). Yet anthropologist Michele Friedner cautions against romanticizing the potentialities of becoming. Drawing from her work on cochlear implantation, she writes, "While I appreciate this (hopeful) analytic attention to becoming, I am concerned that . . . we are seeing a narrowing or contraction, because it is indeed increasingly possible—through biotechnologies such as cochlear implantation—to become normal" (2022b, 165). Currently, and in contrast to deafness, biotechnologies play a more limited role in making Down syndrome and are primarily felt through the consequences of prenatal testing. The expanding capacities of gene-editing technologies, however, raise questions about the future possibilities—and limitations—of "becoming" with Down syndrome. When sutured to expectations of becoming *something*, becoming may easily reinforce hegemonic constructions of normal, standard, desirable, or "better."[2]

Acceptance did not portend clear outcomes for being or becoming. Instead it presented Down syndrome families, individuals, and outside parties with conflicting "best goods" at different moments (Mattingly 2014a, 2014b). Across its many possible permutations, however, acceptance created space to inhabit and dwell in the world with Down syndrome and alongside people with Down syndrome.[3] An inherently intersubjective and often interworldly project (Friedner 2020), acceptance made strong claims on mothers and on "the horizons of possibility, intersubjectivity, and self-reflection that motherhood invites" (Willen 2014, 86). This did not lead to agreements between mothers and children—or the many other actors I have introduced throughout this book—on *how* to struggle for acceptance or to what ends. But it nevertheless coded an "existential imperative" to *be*-in-the-world and be-with Down syndrome.

KINSHIP FUTURES YET TO COME

Ethnography offers snippets of lives lived and lost. The kinship futures outlined in this book appeared at a specific historical juncture—the mid-2010s. Hana's warning that "it's not always the older generation that dies first" proved unimaginably prescient as the cataclysm of COVID-19 engulfed the world. I witnessed the virus's initial spread from Amman, having started (what was supposed to be) a five-month research fellowship in January 2020. By the time the government confirmed Jordan's first official case of COVID-19 on March 2, 2020, I had already paused my preliminary fieldwork; the risks of entering and exiting the clinical settings where I hoped to conduct ethnographic research had become obviously unacceptable.

On March 14, three days after the World Health Organization declared a global pandemic, the government announced its plans to close all schools, nonessential businesses, and borders. On March 18, I traded Jordan's relative safety for the pandemonium spreading across the United States. Three days later, King Abdullah II announced a total curfew that was reinforced by the military and police, at least in the capital. By March 25 the government began allowing limited movement on foot, but the curfew (in effect from 6:00 P.M.–10:00 A.M.) persisted for months. These extraordinarily aggressive measures reflected how "Jordan was coercively well-equipped to institute a lockdown, while being structurally ill-equipped to deal with a large outbreak" (Jensehaugen 2020).

Given the immunological vulnerabilities precipitated by Down syndrome, especially with regard to respiratory illnesses (Espinosa 2020), fear of infection proved well-founded. Early data quickly confirmed that people with Down syndrome were at higher risk for hospitalization and experienced more severe outcomes (Clift et al. 2021; Malle et al. 2020, 2021). The imperative to "stay at home" (*khalik bil-bayt*) felt cruelly ironic to many families, given that they measured the struggle for acceptance partly in terms of getting their children out of the house and into society.[4] In addition to worrying about immunocompromised children, parents wrestled with their own vulnerability. The more distant shores of mortality surged closer, and disability cliffs that had loomed safely at further remove arrived prematurely on the doorstep.

As we kept in touch over WhatsApp, my interlocutors lamented failing small businesses, bemoaned the "disaster" of distance learning, and struggled to cope with the crushing boredom of lockdown. They also worried about rising family tensions, especially with husbands atypically confined to the home. Toward the end of March 2021, during Jordan's second major wave, my Facebook feed flooded with announcements that the government would begin prioritizing vaccine access for disabled people. The result of grassroots efforts by disabled persons organizations, family advocates, and the Higher Council for the Rights of Persons with Disabilities (HCD), the campaign elicited expressions of gratitude and enthusiasm alongside consternation from vaccine skeptics. The HCD and other public accounts spent the next few weeks documenting their efforts on social media. The photos and videos offered a welcome respite from the otherwise steady stream of prayer requests for the sick and death announcements made on behalf of those who had succumbed to the virus.

When I returned in spring 2023, nearly three years to the day after my chaotic departure, everyone looked older. My newly established gray streaks raised eyebrows among friends. I finally retrieved the prescription sunglasses I had accidentally left at Reem's house in March 2020 and marveled at her children's transition to fully fledged teenagers who towered over me. I visited Umm Farha on the fringes of southwest Amman, where urban sprawl gives way to open fields and steep valleys. As she maneuvered an unfamiliar road back to the city center, I nervously eyed two large dogs perched on the rocky cliffs bordering our asphalt trajectory. While conflicts with stray dogs were not new (McClellan 2019), Amman was on edge after several severe attacks, and one young boy died from a postinjury infection shortly after my arrival.

Those menacing canine silhouettes embodied a post-COVID world, supposedly returning to "normal" but clearly still gone awry. Some of the families introduced in this book emerged relatively unscathed from the pandemic's devastation (whose economic dimensions were exacerbated by Jordan's shutdown and the limited impact of worker protections on its highly informalized work force). Others were less fortunate. The absence of key parents and children whom I would otherwise have sought to visit filled my return with pangs of incomplete mourning. COVID-19 possessed a fearsome capacity to unmake Down syndrome—and everything else—through epidemiological and social costs that amplify how kinship functions as a conduit for life-threatening risk and a mechanism for life-saving protection. COVID-19 rearranged timelines of life, death, and disability (and book writing) in profound ways. Now other crises, as near as Occupied Palestine and as distant as the United States, bear more heavily on imaginable kinship futures.

This book offers an account of how kinship futures—hopes, fears, and claims forged through family relations and roles—loop back to make Down syndrome in Jordan's (no longer) present. Yet kinship futures are equally about the past.

They emerge from specific histories—of family, land, displacement, and dispossession—and converge in what people experience as "now." The alchemy of making Down syndrome unfolds at the nexus of global disability discourses and local realities, with the latter always already entangled in "the global." In Jordan, these include intensifying demographic pressures, worsening economic conditions, and political crises that both destabilize and reconstitute kinship futures, even threatening to erase them entirely.[5] As people with Down syndrome live longer and healthier lives on an increasingly unstable and inhospitable planet, they will challenge families, neighbors, and societies to engage in new projects of acceptance. And while no one can know what comes next, kinship (and other) futures will continue to make and remake Down syndrome in ways yet to be seen.

ACKNOWLEDGMENTS

This book is the culmination of several years of twists and turns, of starts and stops (more than I ever anticipated). First and foremost, my gratitude goes to my interlocutors. Some I crossed paths with only briefly or intermittently, while others allowed me into their lives and their homes with remarkable kindness and hospitality. I have used pseudonyms in place of their names to try and provide them and their families privacy.

Everyone needs friends whom they can text with panicked questions about transliteration, interspersed with more general expressions of existential dread. Susan MacDougall has likely read every word I have ever written, in one form or another. She is endlessly generous with her time and gentle with her feedback, and I have been more than fortunate to benefit from her unparalleled ethnographic sensibility. Rayya El Zein's critical insight and steely resilience were always there to remind me that giving up was not an option. Eda Pepi's hospitality and gift for storytelling provided a life raft on more than one occasion when I found myself nearly drowning.

In the many years spent revising my dissertation into its current form, Jess Newman and Nama Khalil offered patient readings and unfailing moral support while nurturing their own busy lives and blossoming careers. Geoffrey Hughes, Bridget Guarasci, Kate MacClellan, Allison Mickel, Jose Martinez, and Sarah Tobin are colleagues I see far too infrequently, and I am always grateful when we cross paths. In the chaos of winter/early spring 2020, Barbara Porter, Helen Ayyoub, Jackie Salzinger, Jessica Herland, and Starling Carter provided precious companionship and solidarity in Amman. My wonderful Madaba hosts have always welcomed me and humored my mostly unannounced arrivals on their doorstep.

Among a vibrant and growing community of disability anthropologists, I owe an immense debt to Michele Friedner and Cassandra Hartblay for their ceaseless support and their careful engagement with my work and my life. Tyler Zoanni, Patrick McKearney, Helena Fietz, Eliza Williamson, Shruti Vaidya, and Timothy Loh have proven important intellectual interlocutors and patient readers. I have also benefited from two interdisciplinary disability/SWANA studies panels convened by Sara Scalenghe, which allowed me to connect with wonderful scholars like Beverly Tsacoyianis, Halla Atallah, and Shahd Alshammari. Far too brief but no less impactful exchanges with Ayo Wahlberg, Zhiying Ma, Ana Vinea, Lamia Moghnieh, Ellen Rubenstein, and Jane Saffitz also bear their imprint on my thinking.

Fida Adely, Farha Ghannam, Tine Gammeltoft, and Faye Ginsburg graciously participated in a manuscript workshop in the winter of 2024, giving me some faith that the book could become a book. I especially appreciate Fida's continued support, ever since serving as the esteemed discussant on a 2015 American Anthropological Association panel of (then) graduate student anthropologists working in and on Jordan. Andrew Shryock, Kriszti Fehervary, and Elizabeth Roberts have remained consistent cheerleaders from Ann Arbor. Going further into the past, Lara Deeb and Pardis Mahdavi set me on the path I have now been traveling since 2007.

My precious Mountain West crew—Allison Caine, Anna Antoniou, and Bree Doering—have kept me grounded since moving to Colorado. I am not sure how Alli finds the time and energy to cheerlead me through this process, and I eagerly await the day when Anna and I again become neighbors. Emma Bunkley's arrival at CU Denver offered a rare moment of the stars aligning in my favor. Emily Hammad Mrig remains an inspiration for her tenacity and unparalleled ability to multitask in scholarly pursuits and in life. Elizabeth Johnson always lent a sympathetic ear and sound perspective. I would be remiss not to thank my colleagues and students in the Anthropology Department at the University of Colorado Denver, as we have weathered intense global, national, and institutional challenges with levity and compassion.

Funding sources for this book (and the dissertation it draws from) include the Fulbright U.S. Student Program, the University of Michigan (including the Rackham School for Graduate Studies, the Department of Anthropology, the International Institute, and the Center for the Education of Women), Foreign Language and Area Studies Arabic fellowships, a postdoctoral fellowship through the American Center of Research/National Endowment for the Humanities (in Jordan), and a Wenner Gren Hunt Postdoctoral Fellowship. Portions of chapter 6 were previously published in the article "Kinship, Connective Care, and Disability in Jordan," published in *Medical Anthropology*, vol. 40, issue 2, pages 116–128.

Without Lenore Manderson, there would be no book. Her persistence, insights, and support have made it possible for this project to reach its long-awaited conclusion. Similarly, Micha Radher's keen editorial eye and boundless empathy have left me with debts that I cannot repay.

I am wildly appreciative that my parents, Barbara and Peter, and my sister Lauren (and Ryan, Cooper, and Carson) have never doubted me or my choices (at least out loud) And to Travis and our most faithful nonhuman companions (present and passed), thank you for remaining by my side as I have perpetually unraveled and tried to put myself back together again.

Finally, the wisdom, patience, and generosity of the women I call Umm Farha and Reem matter more than they could know or I could ever hope to convey. Nurturing friendship across the devastation wrought by U.S. empire has never been easy, but these past few years have been truly devastating. I am thankful that our capacity for human connection endures across the gross inequalities and injustices that shape our lives and (kinship) futures yet to come. May they be more equitable and more just.

NOTES

CHAPTER 1   DOWN SYNDROME AND KINSHIP FUTURES

1. When using my own narrative voice, I mostly employ identity-first language ("disabled children"; "disabled person"). When directly translating or transliterating, I preserve my interlocutors' phrasings, which typically took a "person-first" construction. In English-language contexts, the political stakes of person-first versus disability-first language continue to generate intense discussion and disagreement (Brown 2011; Dunn and Andrews 2015). In Jordan, I encountered a different set of terminological disagreements and transformations (see chapter 2).

2. Some people consider this teknonym old-fashioned or déclassé, but it was common among the families I met, and it gestures to how kinship—and especially parenthood—provides critical coordinates for navigating Jordanian social and moral worlds. In the traditional formula (known in Arabic as *kunya*), parents assume the name of their oldest child, with a firstborn son taking precedence over daughters. In practice, however, parents may be identified more situationally. For example, while many people referred to one of my closest interlocutors, Umm Farha, by the name of her oldest son, Ahmed, others called her Umm Farha because Farha's Down syndrome precipitated her entry into disability advocacy. To minimize reader confusion, I refer to parents by the pseudonym of their child with Down syndrome (or child who was otherwise intellectually disabled) rather than using the more conventional practices of adopting the name of one's firstborn child or eldest son.

3. In Jordan these interdependencies are embedded in the highest levels of government and industry, where a core network of families connected by descent, marriage, and other strategic partnerships benefit from the monarchy's relentless pursuit of neoliberal reforms (Hourani 2014; Martínez 2017; Ryan 2011; Yom 2015).

4. Grounded in cultural and disability studies, crip theory examines how a "system of compulsory able-bodiedness, which in a sense produces disability, is thoroughly interwoven with the system of compulsory sexuality that produces queerness" (McRuer 2006, 2).

5. Arseli Dokumacı describes her interlocutors with rheumatoid arthritis as "noncrips" (2023, 12) because many did not identify as crip and were unfamiliar with the politics informing the term. She cautions that crip "exposure and familiarity may not be available to subjects whose subjection occurs outside North American discourses, geographies, and histories from which identity politics (and its subsequent critiques) have emerged" (12).

6. Intellectually disabled self-advocates and allies have spent decades organizing against "the R-word" (for examples, see statements by the Special Olympics, The Arc, and the Autistic Self Advocacy Network). To honor that advocacy, I have chosen to mask the term with a "-." The Arabic equivalent, *takhalluf* (adjective: *mutakhalluf*), provoked different reactions among my interlocutors. Some considered the term akin to a slur, while others considered it outdated and medically inaccurate but not necessarily offensive.

7. In a minority percentage of cases (widely cited rates range from approximately 3–5%), Down syndrome occurs due to translocation, which means that the extra chromosome 21 attaches itself to another chromosome. An unaffected parent can be a carrier for a translocated chromosome 21, but translocation can also occur during cell development. No differences can be discerned in trisomy versus translocation Down syndrome.

8. An equally small number of Down syndrome cases (approximately 2–5%) are considered *mosaic*, which means that due to the timing of cell division, some of the body's cells acquire a third chromosome 21 but others do not. There is limited research on whether and how mosaicism results in different presentations of Down syndrome (see the International Mosaic Down Syndrome Association for more information).

9. "Making" departs from the strictly social model of disability (Oliver 1990; UPIAS 1976) that emphasizes how social structures and norms transmute differences of functional capacity (impairment) into sustained and systemic disadvantage (disability). An anchor for disability rights movements and legislation around the world, the social model informs Jordan's major disability law, as well as the human rights and development paradigms that circulate through Jordanian civil society and shape how people imagine and claim disability (see chapter 2). Yet the model cannot so easily account for disability's diverse lived realities or political multiplicities. In response to its limitations, scholars in critical disability studies have drawn on feminist, critical race, and decolonial theory to highlight the sociality of embodiment and the racialized politics of impairment that unequally distribute likelihoods of becoming disabled (Annamma 2018; Corker 2001; Erevelles 2011; Goodley et al. 2012; Goodley 2013; Grech and Soldatic 2016; Meekosha and Soldatic 2011). I build on their critical departures by bringing this intersectional framework together with an "ethnographic sensibility" that unsettles Global North–centric historical and political genealogies of disability (Aciksoz 2019; Friedner 2015, 2022a; Friedner and Zoanni 2018; Ingstad and Reynolds Whyte 1995; McGranahan 2018; Nakamura 2013; Phillips 2010).

10. I use descriptions of both Middle East and North Africa (MENA) and Southwest Asia and North Africa (SWANA) in this book. My interlocutors used the Arabic phrase for the Middle East (al-Sharq al-Awsat) as a geographical and identity category. The shift from MENA to SWANA reflects ongoing attempts to decolonize the former (see Bishara 2023). There is one context where I have seen (S)WANA used *in* Jordan. The West Asia North Africa Institute, chaired by His Royal Highness Prince El Hassan bin Talal (brother of King Abdullah II), notes on its website that the region known as the Middle East is only east "from the perspective of Europe." The organization's intentional use of WANA "advocates for a definition of the region less rooted in political geography, but rather in human geography." The acronym does not translate to Arabic, however, which gestures at the complexities of audience.

11. The women migrants who usually provide care for impaired or aging Jordanians travel from the Philippines, Ethiopia, or Sri Lanka and live in their employers' homes. The *kafala* system that structures labor migration in Jordan (and across much of the SWANA region) makes residence in a family home obligatory for some categories of workers (Nasri 2017).

12. "Women nationals can confer their nationality to their children only in special circumstances, such as where the father's nationality is unknown, the father is stateless, or where the father's filiation is not established" (ESCWA 2018b, 20).

13. Sharia courts deal with PSL-related topics for the country's Muslim majority, while church law and ecclesiastical courts manage these same issues for the Christian minority, who account for approximately 2–3 percent of the population. Article 1086 of the kingdom's civil code obligates Jordanians of all faiths to follow Sharia law when it comes to the distribution of inheritance; this usually means that daughters receive only half of the assets distributed to sons. In the absence of sons, a portion of the inheritance is distributed to uncles or male cousins. In practice, both Muslim and Christian families pressure women to surrender their entire inheritance to male relatives. While the leaders of Jordan's Christian denominations submitted a proposal in spring 2023 that would guarantee equal distribution between men and women, it has yet to be approved by the government and faces opposition from some men in Christian communities (Kuttab 2023).

14. Unmarried women under the age of forty can be reported to local authorities for "absences" from the home (HRW 2023; Amnesty International 2019). A guardian's consent is legally required for the first marriage of any woman under thirty. In cases of divorce, mothers usually receive custody (*hadana*) but not guardianship; they are also legally obligated to relinquish custody if they choose to remarry. While a child's father is de facto awarded guardianship, this requirement transfers to any male relative or the court in a father's absence. The court can deprive a father or grandfather of guardianship if they are proven to be incompetent, and a mother can obtain guardianship in exceptional cases if she can prove that both the father and paternal grandfather should not be granted this right (Musawah 2017).

15. The importance of marriage can be gleaned from the high marriage rates present throughout the kingdom: 82.7 percent of women and 96.5 percent of men aged forty-five to forty-nine are married (DOS and ICF 2023).

16. These data come from the most recent (2023) Population and Family Health Survey.

17. Despite the rising age at first marriage, dating remains highly regulated if not forbidden, and young people resort to more surreptitious channels for flirting and socializing (Kaya 2009). Even elite families who otherwise embrace social norms and traditions associated with "the West" balk at the practice of cohabitation outside wedlock. The criminalization of extramarital sex, although not widely enforced, reinforces this taboo.

18. Most of Amman's informal settlements were built by Palestinian refugees in the 1950s and 1960s and perch on the edges of Amman's many hills (*jabals*) and down into its floodable valley zones (*wadis*). Several of Amman's oldest neighborhoods take the preface of Jabal, but "Jabal Ahmar" is a pseudonym.

19. During my fieldwork, the rise of the Islamic State, known by its Arabic acronym of Daesh, was a topic of serious concern and political conflict, a limitless source of cultural commentary and satire, and grounds for a dramatic national loss. In January 2015, ISIS militants captured, imprisoned, and subsequently burned alive the twenty-six-year-old Jordanian pilot Muath Al-Kasasbeh. The brutal killing horrified the country and intensified local scrutiny of Jordan's military involvement in the Syrian crisis.

20. The terms "Bedouin" and "tribal" are not synonymous, although their conflation plays an important role in Jordanian national narratives (Adely 2012a; Massad 2001; Watkins 2014; Wilson 1990). Contemporary associations with "tribe" and "tribal" often prove unhelpful for understanding how associations of kin, clan, and tribe shape daily life and politics in Jordan. The Circassians (and later Chechens) who welcomed Emir Abdullah to the sparsely populated and newly established farmlands of Amman made their way to the region as refugees fleeing Tsarist Russian expansion and the Ottoman-Balkan wars. They were resettled by Ottoman authorities through several waves of migration between 1878 and 1906 (Shami 2009).

21. The plan called for expropriating over half of mandate Palestine to the Jewish population, who comprised less than one-third of the population and owned less than 7 percent of the land (Khalidi 1997).

22. Ten Palestinian refugee camps and three (official) Syrian refugee camps are located in Jordan. Most Gazan refugees from the Six-Day War of 1967 live in the Jerash camp, located in the northern governorate of Jerash. Unlike those displaced in 1948, this later wave of Gazan refugees did not receive Jordanian citizenship. This means that they do not have social security numbers, cannot enroll their children in public schools, and do not qualify for public health care. They also face severe restrictions on working (Pérez 2021, 2024).

23. Disputed terrorism accusations leveled against UNRWA by Israel in 2023, after the October 7 Hamas attacks, dealt a severe blow to the organizations's already deteriorating fiscal stability and functionality. Despite the dramatic impact of these allegations, serious doubts remain about the validity of Israel's evidence (Noestlinger and Baczynska 2024; Nichols and

Perry 2024). A report by the National Intelligence Council noted that it "assessed with 'low confidence' that a handful of staff had participated in the attack, indicating that it considered the accusations to be credible though it could not independently confirm their veracity" (Guardian Staff 2024). This assessment contradicts Secretary of State Anthony Blinken's description of the accusations as "highly, highly credible" (Guardian Staff 2024). As of July 2024, Australia, Austria, Canada, Estonia, Finland, Germany, Iceland, Italy, Japan, Latvia, Lithuania, Romania, and Sweden restored funding to the UNRWA; France, Denmark, Switzerland, New Zealand, and the European Union never stopped payments; the United States and United Kingdom remain conspicuous outliers (HRW 2024). For more context on Israel's campaign against UNRWA, which long precedes the attacks of October 7, see the extensive coverage by Jadaliyya.

24. Most Palestinians in Jordan are Jordanian citizens who hold Jordanian passports. Gazan refugees, however, remain stateless (see note 22). After 1988, Jordan changed its policy toward Palestinians living in the West Bank, granting "temporary passports" that function as travel documents but lack the "national number" required to access the privileges of Jordanian citizenship (Gabbay 2014; HRW 2010). Palestinians living in the Occupied Palestinian Territory (West Bank and Gaza) are issued green identification cards by the Israeli military, while those born in East Jerusalem and Israel are issued blue identification cards. The Palestinian Authority has been able to issue passports for residents of the Occupied Territory since the Oslo Accords, but individuals must receive permission from Israeli authorities to travel abroad, to travel from Gaza to the West Bank (which is only granted for humanitarian medical reasons), or to travel from the West Bank to Gaza (which requires a pledge to settle permanently in Gaza).

25. The number of Syrians counted in Jordan's 2015 census (1,265,514) remains contested (Turner 2023, 883; see also Lenner 2020, 286), as it considerably exceeded the total number of refugees *registered* with the U.N. High Commission on Refugees at that time. The vast majority of displaced Syrians live in urban areas rather than refugee camps (UNHCR 2025).

26. To preserve a greater degree of anonymity, I do not always explicitly identify families as Syrian or Iraqi, since having a child with Down syndrome amplifies their identifiability in Amman's compressed social networks.

27. As discussed in note 20, the word "tribal" comes with heavy analytical baggage (in Jordan and elsewhere). Yet Jordanians of diverse backgrounds used this adjective, as well as the noun of tribalism, to describe and differentiate various communal and ethnic dynamics. This included Jordanians of Palestinian descent describing "East Bank" Jordanians as more influenced by the power of "tribal" structures and affiliations.

28. When self-advocate Frank Stephens testified in front of the U.S. Congress in 2017, translations of his speech subsequently made their way across my Arabic-language Facebook feed. His was one of the many "success stories" (*qisas najah*) that circulate through Arabic-language and Jordan-specific social media as examples of how to make and live with Down syndrome (even so, horror stories—of neglect, abandonment, abuse—circulate as well).

29. While residents of Amman might be less likely to identify themselves as "Ammani," I follow the anthropologist Sarah Tobin (2016) in using the term to highlight the capital's specific political and cultural dynamics, its complexity and diversity notwithstanding.

30. In articulating this approach, I find helpful parallels with Tey Meadows's methodological discussion around their decision *not* to interview children while studying the emergent category of "transgender children" (2018).

31. This might be surprising to a consumer of Jordanian public talk shows, which often feature children and adults with Down syndrome talking directly with audiences about their lives. But participants in these productions rarely, if ever, attend or engage without parents or siblings accompanying them (or, in some cases, teachers and coaches). Their presence may be subtle, but it remains significant to dynamics of supervision and surveillance.

CHAPTER 2   DISABILITY IMAGINARIES

1. *'Ayb* literally translates to "fault" or "defect" (Wehr 1993). Colloquially and semantically, however, "'ayb references that which is deemed culturally, morally or socially shameful but not forbidden" (Odgaard 2022, 46). I will return to questions and tensions of *'ayb* in chapter 3.

2. Throughout this chapter, I use "imaginary" in the indefinite or plural to foreground "people's imaginaries. This person-centered approach recognizes the importance of learned cultural understandings but does not take 'culture' to be a fixed entity assumed to be held in common by a geographically bounded or self-identified group" (Strauss 2006, 323).

3. I understand disability imaginaries to function differently from "cripwashing," a phenomenon whereby a government invokes performances of disability rights to undermine other targeted civil liberties (Moscoso and Platero 2017). Disability imaginaries also depart from the "ablenationalism" described by David Mitchell and Sharon Snyder because disability imaginaries emphasize barriers of supposed cultural backwardness and lack of development (Mitchell 2015; Snyder and Mitchell 2010).

4. English-language coverage of the documentary refers to it as *Jordan's Secret Shame*. Neither Arabic media coverage nor the film itself uses this title (*AlBawaba* 2012; *Amman Net* 2012; BBC Arabic 2012).

5. Elsewhere in the Levant, mental institutions and asylums became well-established in local landscapes of healing and health governance during the first quarter of the twentieth century (Abi-Rached 2020; Moghnieh 2022; Tsacoyianis 2021). Presumably, intellectually and developmentally disabled people would have been admitted to these sites as patients. Jordan's only public psychiatric hospital, formerly the Fuheis Psychiatric Hospital and now the National Center for Mental Health, was built in 1987. Al Rashid Hospital, the country's first private psychiatric hospital, opened in 1996. Little has been written about either. Given their relatively recent establishment, it is unclear how contemporary distinctions between intellectual, developmental, and psychiatric disability might affect their admission policies.

6. An alternative rendering of *haki fadi* would be "bullshit" (Martínez 2022, 137).

7. The Human Rights Watch report *Living in Chains* (2020) focuses on the global practice of shackling persons living with "psychosocial disabilities." It does not, however, address the legibility of the term "psychosocial disabilities" in local contexts. Many of the examples provided instead describe the shackling experienced by people with "perceived mental health conditions *or* intellectual disabilities" (2020, 10; my emphasis). Anecdotally, the framework of psychiatric and mental *illness* seemed more popular than psychiatric or psychosocial *disability*, both in academic literature and in everyday use (see, for example, Vinea 2023). For ethnographically driven discussions of confinement and disability in the context of East Asia, see work by Zhiying Ma (2020) and Karen Nakamura (2013).

8. The *Global Report on Health Equity for Persons with Disabilities* (WHO 2022) estimates a global disability prevalence rate of 16 percent, an increase of 1 percent from the 2011 *Global Report*. The report highlights the same north–south disparity first quantified in 2011, placing disability prevalence for high-income countries at 21.2 percent and the prevalence for low-income countries dropping to 12.8 percent (23). The report goes into considerable detail explaining its updated methodology (WHO 2022, 22–24). Concerning prevalence estimates, developed countries consistently report higher rates of disability than developing countries, and survey instruments typically result in higher rates than census data collected from the same populations (Mont 2007). For example, while the Centers for Disease Control and Prevention (2024b) estimates that 28.7 percent of Americans have some type of disability, census figures put disability prevalence at 13 percent of the noninstitutionalized population (Leppert and Schaeffer 2023).

9. Linguistic and cultural issues with translating survey instruments have been especially well examined in relation to Likert scales (Flaskerud 1988; Lee et al. 2002; Summers et al. 2019).

10. In the CRPD's official Arabic translation, this definition reads as follows: ويشمل مصطلح "الأشخاص ذوي الإعاقة" كـل مـن يعـانون من عاهات طويلة الأجل بدنيـة أو عقليـة أو ذهنيـة أو حـسية. This translation is posted on the website of the U.N.'s Department of Economic and Social Affairs.

11. The root letters of this verb are *ayn, waw,* and *qaf.*

12. A wide variety of characteristics and conditions fell under the label of *'ahat,* including "blindness, deafness and paraplegia; diseases like leprosy and halitosis; temporary ailments like ophthalmia and jaundice; extraordinary physical features like blue eyes, crossed eyes, flat noses, black skin, baldness, hunched backs, lisps and thin beards" (Richardson 2012, 6).

13. The etiologies of impairment that Scalenghe details through Ottoman archival sources offer tentative insights into how those with a condition like Down syndrome might have lived during earlier historical periods. While humoral theories of imbalance provided the basis for more flexible designations, "idiocy" (*'ataha*) conveyed a sense of permanence. It was assigned to those with congenital or early childhood impairments, and it resulted in persistent marginalization (Scalenghe 2014, 89).

14. Both Richardson (2012) and Scalenghe (2014) criticize the assumption that disabled people's presently marginalized status reflects either historical continuity or religious justification. My interlocutors also commented on the overlaps and differences between the Qur'anic terms associated with blindness and deafness and contemporary disability language. In the Qur'an, blindness and deafness are deployed as metaphors for states of being of those who do not heed the word of God, but the words used to describe these moral failures differ from those used by Arabic speakers of the time to describe the physiological conditions of blindness or deafness (Bazna and Hatab 2005). Given these discrepancies of terminology, scholars argue that the Qur'an's negative descriptions of deafness and blindness should be understood as judgments of nonbelievers or those who willfully ignore the word of God rather than of people with vision or hearing impairments (Bazna and Hatab 2005; Ghaly 2016).

15. Sara Scalenghe and I have communicated privately about whether the term *mongholi* might first have traveled to Jordan through British colonial missionary medical activities.

16. Many of my interlocutors perceived *mongholi* as an inappropriate and inaccurate confusion of national and ethnic identities. Connotations of stupid (*habla*) and crazy (*majnun*) further amplified opposition to the term, but they did not explicitly describe it as racist (*'unsuri*) or connect these qualities to racialized categories and frameworks.

17. Patient-based collectives elsewhere recognized under the mantle of "biosociality" (Rabinow 2005) have not emerged as swiftly in the SWANA region (Beaudevin 2013). Biosociality seems ill-suited to capture the emotionally charged connections that Down syndrome families—and especially mothers—developed with each other, especially given their diminished interest in or capacity to organize politically and make claims on the state. The anthropologist Elizabeth Roberts has elsewhere cautioned that "the concept should not be applied to every social grouping formed around a biological identity or disease status. Biosociality involves an empirically traceable reimagining of the nature of the social and the biological in the face of new biomedical and genetic knowledge or diagnostic technologies" (2008, 81).

18. In *Cognitive Disability and Its Challenge to Moral Philosophy* (2010, 1), the philosophers Licia Carlson and Eve Feder Kittay address the issue of language on the first page of the book. They write: "We've chosen the term 'cognitive disability,' under which we include conditions like autism, dementia, Alzheimer's, and mental r-tardation, rather than 'intellectual disability.' The former is broader. Also, some forms of cognitive disability do not imply diminished intel-

lectual capacity (e.g., autism)." Many readers, however, would reject Carlson and Kittay's use of what Down syndrome communities in North America refer to as the "r-word."

19. In her work with members of an Egyptian Sufi order, the anthropologist Amira Mittermaier recalls the doubts that emerged after a toddler's dream foreshadowed the death of their community's religious leader. They did not question the capacity of dreams to portend future events, but the age status of the dream's recipient raised concerns. "According to all schools of Islamic law," Mittermaier writes, "a child of that age lacks reason ('aql), and according to many Egyptians I know, children should not always be believed because they tend to make up things" (Mittermaier 2012, 248). From the perspective of Islamic law, however (which forms an important backdrop for Jordanian laws), diminished 'aql does not automatically reduce an individual to the status of a minor (Ghaly 2019).

20. A *Say/Don't Say* language guide available on the Higher Council on the Rights of Persons with Disabilities'(Alazzeh, n.d.) mentions 'aql only when discussing the "Don't Say" phrase of *mutakhallaf 'aqliyyan* (mentally r-tarded). The sheet replaces this with "a person with a disability" that is *dhihniyya* in nature. The corresponding explanation, however, focuses on the unacceptability of the word "r-tardation" (*takhalluf*) rather than on their substitution of *'aql* with *dhihn*. While in the field, and later on social media, I queried native Arabic speakers about how they perceived both terms. Many found it challenging to articulate the differences between them, and only some described them as meaningfully distinct.

21. While the issue of person-first or identity-first language provokes considerable disagreement in English-language contexts (Dunn and Andrews 2015; Gernsbacher 2017), it did not carry the same gravity in Jordan. This may reflect the influence of cultural context and grammatical structures.

22. Law No. 20 of 2017 tasked the Ministry of Education (MOE) with creating its own standards for educational diagnosis. In its 2018–2022 strategy plan, the MOE set the goal for itself of creating three diagnostic centers by 2023, which would serve students in north, central, and south Jordan, as well as two mobile clinics for students living in refugee camps.

23. The Zeids belong to the Iraqi branch of the Hashemite family. Prince Ra'ed's wife, Princess Majda, cofounded and previously served as the president of the Al-Hussein Society.

24. In 2010 the Higher Council published a registry identifying 290 organizations and 12 sports clubs focused on disability across the kingdom, with just under half located in the capital. The registry describes these organizations as institutions/foundations (*mu'assasat*), which does not correspond to any of the designations outlined in the Law on Societies (see note 25). "Institutions/foundations" might correspond most closely with "closed societies" according to the Law on Society's definitions. The majority of organizations listed in the registry, however, self-identified as charitable and mission-driven, with their names including the word "society" (*jama'iyya*).

25. Baylouny (2006) cautions against interpreting family societies as straightforward reflections of preexisting kin ties or structures. To the contrary, in these associations kin ties "are actively constructed, often entailing the recruitment of 'new' family members. Family genealogies have been rewritten, sometimes reaching back over a thousand years, to redefine the present kin group. Others split off from the larger group to create a smaller definition of family" (350).

26. Most of these organizations operate under the jurisdiction of the Law on Societies No. 51 of 2008 and its 2009 amendments. The law differentiates between three categories of societies (*jama'iyyat*): societies, closed societies, and private societies (the distinctions between them pertain to the number of required members and funding structures).

27. Any foreign donation must receive approval from the Ministry of Planning and International Cooperation while closed societies can, by definition, only receive funding from members.

28. For more on information, see the World Down Syndrome Day website, https://www
.worlddownsyndromeday.org/about-wdsd.

29. According to data from the 2009 census, 1 percent of primary school–aged children were
not enrolled in school (with equal gender parity). This rate worsens over time, however, with
10 percent of girls out of school in secondary school—and 15 percent of boys (FHI 360 and
EPDC 2018).

30. According to a 2017–2018 survey conducted by the Department of Statistics, 40 percent
of Jordanian households' yearly expenditures fell between 5,000 and 10,000 dinar, with an
additional 8.8 percent falling below 5,000 dinar per year (*Jordan Times* 2018).

31. Jordan's main approach to inclusive education during my fieldwork relied on the establishment of "resource rooms," which remain prominent throughout the kingdom today. Most
parents and specialists perceived resource rooms negatively for a variety of reasons. They
often suffer from a lack of coordination and cooperation between the resource room teacher
and the general education teacher, as well as overcrowding and inadequate teacher training
(Al Khatib and Al Khatib 2008; Amr 2011). More foundationally, resource rooms do not com-
ply with the definition of inclusive education outlined in Jordan's older or newer Disability
Rights Law, nor with the CRPD (Alodat et al. 2014). These issues have received consistent
attention in unpublished Arabic-language dissertations and master's theses by students at Jordanian universities, many supervised by Dr. Jamal Al-Khatib at the University of Jordan.
Other unpublished Arabic-language reports are housed in the Ministry of Education.

32. These numbers point to issues with data collection and diagnostic inconsistency, as
they are significantly lower than the figures collected ten years prior. In 2007, Al Khatib
and Al Khatib (2008) reported that 511 public school resource rooms served 12,300 children
with disabilities in grades 2 through 6 (109). Given the lack of standardized diagnostic and
evaluation procedures, staff often classify students as having "learning disabilities," and it is
unclear whether this designation overlaps with intellectual and developmental disability.
Occasionally, I met children with intellectual disabilities who *only* attended resource room
classes at a mainstream school via individual arrangements made between school administrators, teachers, and parents. "Shadow teachers" have increased inclusion of students with
disabilities, but individual families may be asked to cover the cost of that teacher's salary.

33. While the literacy rate among youth and adult populations (aged fifteen and over) in Jordan is 99 percent (FHI 360 and EPDC 2018), the illiteracy rate among people with disabilities
continues to exceed 30 percent (DOS 2021).

34. Ironically, neoliberal austerity measures may prove the death knell for a liberal arts education and the Enlightenment principles on which these curriculums rely. One need look no
further than the United States to observe the ongoing assaults on the questionable "useful-
ness" (i.e., market return) of the humanities and (humanistic) social sciences.

CHAPTER 3   AFTERSHOCKS

1. *Ya ukhti* literally means "Oh my sister!" but conveys a more familiar sense of exasperation
or interruption.

2. Why nondisjunction (which causes trisomy of chromosome 21) occurs in this not-at-risk
population remains unclear.

3. During her extensive research on gender and kinship in Zabid, Yemen, anthropologist
Anne Meneley's (2003) interlocutors described shock as the primary cause of *faja'a*, or fright
illness. Meneley's interpretation of faja'a as a modality for Zabidi women to experience and
make sense of gendered vulnerability strongly resonates with how my interlocutors experienced and theorized shock.

4. For a different perspective on shifting configurations of Jordanian kinship and the tensions between nuclear units versus broader kinship groupings, see Geoffrey Hughes's *Affection and Mercy* (2021).

5. The Jordanian Ministry of Health runs Jordan's official disability diagnosis centers. The need for an "official" diagnosis continued to crystallize during my fieldwork, as formal policies were then in development. Even Law No. 20 of 2017 described these procedures as in progress, and they continue to evolve.

6. As discussed in the notes to chapter 1, intellectually disabled self-advocates and allies have spent decades organizing against "the R-word." I recognize that advocacy here by choosing not to reproduce the word used by many doctors and nurses. The Arabic equivalent, *takhalluf* (adj: *mutakhalluf*), provoked various reactions among my interlocutors, which ranged from offense and ambivalence to acceptance. The deployment of *takhalluf* as a counterpoint to ideals of progress, development, and modernity in Jordan (and the SWANA region more broadly) gestures to the entangled notions of individual and societal development that I explore in chapter 4.

7. Advances in medical care have dramatically altered the average life expectancy for people with Down syndrome. The advent of corrective heart surgery, in particular, has reduced the impact of congenital defects for infants and young children. Additionally, therapeutic interventions and the provision of generally better care continue to challenge the assumptions that nondisabled people hold about the potentiality and limits of life with Down syndrome (see chapter 1).

8. Even data from the United States in the early 2000s reveal that a majority of mothers received postnatal diagnoses of Down syndrome (Skotko 2005). The advent of noninvasive prenatal testing (NIPT) technologies, however, has presumably shifted this prevalence.

9. According to Jordan's 2023 *Population and Family Health Survey,* 97 percent of pregnant women received prenatal care from a medical professional, and 99 percent had given birth in a medical facility during the previous five years (DOS and ICF 2023, 149). Over the course of their pregnancies, 64 percent made eight or more antenatal care visits (DOS and ICF 2023, 150). Jordan's caesarean rate stands at 43 percent (DOS and ICF 2023), which exceeds the United States' rate of 32.1 percent and the current global rate of 21 percent (Betran et al. 2021; CDC 2024a).

10. The *Population and Family Health Survey* reports nearly universal coverage for "key antenatal services," which include blood pressure measurements, urine samples, blood samples, and weight measurements, but it does not specify coverage beyond those services (DOS and ICF 2023).

11. Tsipy Ivry's work on prenatal diagnostic technologies has shown this to be the case in Japan (2006, 2010).

12. A study by Abdo et al. (2018) suggest that Jordanian women overwhelmingly support more consistent integration of NIPTs into standard health care services.

13. Religious and legal scholars employ dynamic reasoning to weigh the benefits and risks of new medical technologies. Different understandings of ensoulment—recognized as occurring at either 40, 90, or 120 days after conception—are key to these discussions (Hessini 2007; Rispler-Chaim 2007). Historically, "for abortion before 120 days, various opinions have been expressed which can be summed up into three or four main contentions, viz., unconditionally permissible, permissible in case of having an excuse (*'udhr*), and generally reprehensible and forbidden" (Ghaly 2008). Contemporary scholars largely conform to these positions, but they must address questions raised by the expansion of prenatal diagnostics. Deliberations have focused on the stage of pregnancy at which termination can occur and the kinds of impairments that justify this outcome, as guided by principles of mercy, suffering, and social protection for the mother and family (Ghaly 2008).

14. While most recent literature includes Morocco in this list, anthropologist Jess Newman demonstrates in her forthcoming monograph that this claim perpetuates a misreporting of the actual law, which does not grant exceptions to abortion's criminalization based on fetal anomalies (private communication, 2024).

15. Additionally, hospitals or individual doctors may follow policies that remain unofficial or internal to their places of work.

16. Religious scholars contribute to these efforts by drawing on "longstanding traditions within the Islamic corpus warning against such marriages" (Clarke 2007, 390).

17. At the same time, the preference for consanguineous marriage stems partly from the perception that women are "safer" when their partners are connected to them through ties of kinship.

18. My use of "contagion" here exceeds the contemporary biomedical definition of the term to recognize the broader social and even supernatural "forces that flow and sieve through families" (Meinert and Grøn 2019, 581).

19. The acceptability of this practice appears to be waning, but newer mothers' diagnostic experiences remained variable, reflecting the uneven resources and different clinical cultures found in Jordanian hospitals (Khader et al. 2018).

20. Courts may appoint a divorced or widowed woman as a temporary guardian (HRW 2023, 55).

21. For a discussion of connectivity, kinship, and queerness in Amman, see (Odgaard 2021).

22. This scholarship, influenced by structural functionalist and typological approaches to the SWANA region, used arguments about the "honor-shame" complex as evidence of cultural unity among so-called Mediterranean societies (Peristiany 1965). Subsequent scholars have posed methodological, linguistic, and feminist critiques to challenge these essentialist caricatures of shame and honor (Abu-Lughod 1985, 1986; Coombe 1990; Herzfeld 1980; Wikan 1984), but they persist across domains of social interaction and analysis. Without diminishing anthropology's role in fostering these representational injustices, analytical and ethnographic tensions around shame also appear outside SWANA anthropology. Writing about childhood socialization in China, for example, Heidi Fung describes shame as "the quintessential socio-moral emotion" (1999, 181). She notes, however, that "contemporary Western theorists tend to treat shame negatively and primitively as a problem to be solved or a disease to cure; shame is often associated with children, savages, and neurotics" (Fung 1999, 182).

23. The Arabic-language, Amman-based podcast *Eib*, for example, features a catalogue of over ninety episodes; the program's description reads: "Eib [Arabic for "shame"] showcases everyday stories that are shaped by societal norms and gender roles, or any experiences that are tabooed" (Sowt 2024).

24. Hamamy et al. (2005) interviewed 1,032 individuals attending appointments at the National Center for Diabetes, Endocrinology and Genetics in Amman and stratified their results across three generations: (1) Marriages contracted before 1950, (2) marriages contracted between 1950 and 1979, and (3) marriages contracted between 1980 to date. The rates of consanguineous marriage for generations one, two, and three, respectively, were 23.8, 36.1, and 25.6 percent. Marriages between parallel paternal first cousins decreased from 15.1 to 8.1 percent. The 2012 Jordan "Population and Family Health Services Survey" reported that 35 percent of all recorded marriages were consanguineous (Islam et al. 2018), and this rate dropped to 27.5 percent based on data gathered in the 2018 survey (Islam 2021). The 2023 survey did not report on consanguinity.

25. In their foundational (1992) study, Khoury and Massad calculated Jordan's rate of consanguineous marriage at approximately 50 percent, a number corroborated by the 1990 "Population and Family Health Survey" (Islam et al. 2018).

CHAPTER 4   AMBIVALENT INTERVENTIONS

1. While this frog-leg position is normal in newborns, its persistence past a few months can indicate muscle and joint problems.

2. UNICEF defines early childhood as the period between birth and eight years of age. They note that this is "a critical window of opportunity to shape the trajectory of a child's holistic development and build a foundation for their future" and warn that "when children miss out on this once-in-a-lifetime opportunity, they pay the price in lost potential" (2025). The intended age range for early intervention varies between sources, as do descriptions of Portage's target age range, but zero through six is commonly cited. In practice, these ranges can become more flexible, especially as practitioners account for the impact of late diagnosis or delays in seeking services.

3. Down syndrome is often accompanied by hypotonia, or low muscle tone, which affects developmental milestones like crawling, grasping, walking, and speaking. Structural changes in the shape of the upper jaw can also exacerbate difficulties related to feeding and speech that predispose children and adults to respiratory illnesses. Infants also face increased risk for a mitral valve defect that may require surgical intervention shortly after birth or later in life.

4. While a 2022 Arabic Portage guide available in Jordan (created by the special education expert Dr. Suha Tabbal) uses the translation "early learning" (*al-t'allum al-mubakkir*), available publications and reports (see note 7) usually describe Portage as belonging to the broader category of "early intervention" (*al-tadakhkhul al-mubakkir*).

5. The First Intifada refers to several years (1987–1993) of Palestinian protest and revolt against the violent and unbearable living conditions imposed by Israeli Occupation.

6. Portage's configuration of developmental areas have changed over time, presumably reflecting shifting norms and best practices in the fields of early childhood education and child development. Differences in terminology may also reflect how the guide gets adapted and translated into different languages and settings, as well as which version of the guide is available (it is currently in its third edition).

7. At Al-Nur, mothers attended weekly sessions (or biweekly, monthly, or whatever frequency they could manage) at the society rather than in their homes. Both parents and specialists deemed this arrangement preferable to home visits.

8. Jordan's National Strategy for Persons with Disabilities Phase II Action Plan (2010–2015) prioritized expanding early intervention services across the kingdom. A 2016 report convened by the Higher Council for the Rights of Persons with Disabilities (HCD) identified Portage as the most widely used program in the country, alongside programs or curriculums unique to provider institutions (HCD and Bana Center 2016, 51). This same report identified sixty-four centers offering early intervention services across the country, with thirty-eight located in the capital of Amman (HCD and Bana Center 2016, 46). While a slim majority of private centers offered early intervention (51.9%), most public centers (92.3%) and volunteer centers (85.4%) did not (HCD and Bana Center 2016, 48). Article 19 of Law No. 20 on the Rights of Persons with Disabilities (2017) charged the HCD with working with the Ministry of Education (MOE) to develop standards for accreditation and operating procedures. In 2020 the Ministry of Social Development (MOSD), in collaboration with UNICEF and other partners, released a one-hundred-page Arabic-language guide outlining the standard operational procedures for early intervention (2020). (The challenges of coordinating between the MOE and MOSD are a recurring theme in both academic and on-the-ground narratives.) The HCD aims to integrate early intervention programming into public kindergartens, but families that have knowledge and access tend to start earlier at the "centers" described in the 2016 report.

9. Friedner developed this term through her work with deaf Indian sign language users. She uses it to highlight how people "bring together rights, culture, and God in ways that cannot be accommodated by the empty temporal and secular teleology of human rights discourses" (2019, 410).

10. The ethnographic category of *darrab* shifts away from anthropology's well-established interest in self-cultivation among pious Muslims. By considering embodied and relational modes of cultivation beyond (or at least not reducible to) Islam, I join anthropologists like Julia Elyachar (2011) and Farha Ghannam (2011, 2013), who caution against reducing the ethical and moral worlds inhabited by Muslims in SWANA contexts to those of Islamic discourses and institutions.

11. In her work on gender and modernity in colonial Egypt, the historian Omnia El Shakry argues that *tarbiyya* and *adab* offered nationalist modernizers "resources indigenous to the Islamic discursive tradition that emphasized the proper pedagogy for children, cultivation of the body, and the moral education of the self as essential for the constitutions of a rightly guided Islamic community" (1998, 127–128). These Islamic paradigms complemented and reinforced "modernist disciplining of the body and rationalization of the household" (El Shakry 1998, 128; Kashani-Sabet 2006).

12. Barley soup is associated with the Prophet Muhammad. A hadith recounts that whenever a member of his family would fall sick, he would order the preparation of barley soup and command the ill person to drink (El-Seedi et al. 2019). I thank Nama Khalil for teaching me about this connection.

13. For an analysis of language ideologies and deafness in the Jordanian context, see Loh (2022).

14. See MacDougall (2019) for more on how working-class women navigated friendship and enmity under social conditions widely considered to undermine morality in favor of *maslaha*, or self-interest.

15. Anthropologists have long considered emotions as linguistically mediated cultural constructions that are shaped by social and political context (Lutz and Abu-Lughod 1990; Lutz and White 1986; Rebhun 1994; Scheper-Hughes and Lock 1987).

16. Mothers often described disability as *shi min Allah* (something from God) or *amr Allah* (God's command or decree), or that *Allah hala'u/ha Down* (God created him/her with Down syndrome).

17. As explained in the notes to chapter 1, I honor ethnographic texture while hopefully limiting reader confusion by using a modified teknonym formula that connects parents with the name of their child most proximately discussed in the text. Umm Samira's friends and neighbors would have referred to her as Umm Omar, the name of her oldest son.

18. *Dumur al-'aql* literally translates to "destruction of the mind"; I did not hear people use more medicalized terms for brain (*damagh/mukh*).

19. Jansen's analysis of how *'ajr* can be used to avoid recognizing women's labor as *work* has interesting implications for discussions of care labor. Focusing specifically on midwifery, she argues that "the general religious notion of 'ajr, of earning merit by good deeds done in this life for rewards in the hereafter, when applied in the context of women's work, serves to reclassify this work as a gift. And a gift is responded to with a counter-gift, not with wages" (2004, 16).

20. One of the key hadiths used by Islamic legal scholars in deliberating about the question of capacity is "The pen does not record against [i.e., responsibility is waived for] the sleeper until he awakes, the minor until he matures, and the insane until he regains his sanity" (Ghaly 2019; see also Dols 1992). In discussing rewards and accountability, my interlocutors focused broadly on the question of God's judgment (see chapter 6 for additional discussion of *'ajr*).

21. Amira Mittermaier encountered a similar sentiment among young people participating in community service initiatives in Egypt, who frequently reminded each other that "the poor don't need us; we need the poor. They're our gate to paradise" (2014, 524).

CHAPTER 5   GETTING STUCK

1. The historian Omnia El Shakry offers a comprehensive picture of how "the adolescent" (*al-murahiq*) emerged in postwar Egypt "as a social scientific category of analysis, demarcating the psychological literature from the more popular writings of the mainstream press that addressed 'youth'" (2011, 592). This psychologized model stressed the potentially uncontrollable energies and desires of volatile adolescent subjects, who required the knowledge and expertise of psychology and allied fields to contain them. Shakry's analysis, although derived from research with Egyptian primary sources published in the 1930s, resonates with the contemporary discourses of adolescence that I encountered in Jordan.

2. The Qur'an and hadith also discuss *bulugh* (puberty) as a stage that "signifies the transition into adulthood, during which an individual becomes accountable for their actions" (Hashim 2024, 4). Islamic concepts of social and legal maturity are multidimensional, but biological indicators of puberty play a role in the establishment of bulugh.

3. International development and policy fields have long assessed the SWANA region in terms of a demographic "youth bulge" that poses risks to security, economy, and society—and to ruling regimes (Herrera and Bayat 2010; Swedenburg 2007; Sukarieh 2012). The importance of youth activists in sparking and sustaining the Arab Spring uprisings further solidified perceptions of the power and danger of "the youth" (Singerman 2013). Historians have documented the importance of youth to nationalist and postcolonial movements seeking to achieve independence and modernity for the nation-state (El Shakry 2011; Jacob 2011). Anthropologists have explored how youths navigate religious revivalist movements, whether by cultivating or avoiding the demands of pious subjectivity to which these movements aspire and by tracing how they navigate practices of consumption that define and undermine pious middle-classness (Atia 2013; Deeb and Harb 2013; Schielke 2008, 2009, 2012). (The feminine plural of shabab is *sabaya*, but the latter does not hold the same political connotations.)

4. Here, biomedicine overlaps with an Islamic understanding of puberty as the point of maturity. From the perspective of Islamic law, a mature individual is presumed to possess full mental capacity (*istita'a 'aqliyya*) and the ability to execute two forms of legal capacity (*ahliyya*)—obligation and execution (Ghaly 2019). In this Islamically constructed life course, individuals pass through different stages of accountability for religious obligations and commitments (*taklif*), and these assumed transitions are "meticulously linked to mental capacity" (Ghaly 2019, 260). Maturity serves as the point of full capacity, although theologians and jurists commented extensively on how these presumed transitions could be situationally or permanently disrupted.

5. Kafer (2013) develops her concept of embodied asynchrony by analyzing the legal and bioethical controversies surrounding "the Ashley Treatment," named for the young girl who appears in Washington-based court documents associated with her case only as Ashley X. The Ashley Treatment uses controversial growth attenuation surgeries and chemical regimens to arrest development and puberty in significantly disabled children (for further analyses, see Battles and Manderson 2008; Kittay 2019). Its defenders justify the treatment by mobilizing the specter of a threatening future in which Ashley (and children like her) would otherwise be doomed to a lifetime of pain, discomfort, and eventually institutionalization by family members unable to meet her care needs. The Ashley Treatment represents an extreme intervention, only to be considered (and controversially so) in cases of extensive and profound impairment. I did not encounter discussions of this treatment during my fieldwork, nor would someone with Down syndrome be considered an appropriate candidate.

6. This iconic character, drawn by Palestinian artist Naji Al-Ali, depicts the black-and-white outline of a ten-year-old child who has turned away from viewers, his hands clasped behind his back. He represents a symbol of Palestinian displacement, resistance, and defiance.

7. Disability activists and scholars strongly object to medicalized hierarchies of disability, but my interlocutors frequently used ranks of "severe," "intermediate," and "basic/light"; these classifications were reinforced through the diagnostic process and educational evaluations.

8. I struggled with Umm Lina's dialect, which diverged from the urban Palestinian Jordanian to which I was most accustomed, as well as with the flow of her narrative. When my native-Arabic speaking translator and transcriber assistants worked with this audio, they also struggled to follow Umm Lina's story at certain points in the recording, remarking that her words "didn't make sense" in some places. While I was well practiced in asking interlocutors to slow down or explain unfamiliar terms, I hesitated in this interview, given the intensity of the subject matter and Umm Lina's verbosity.

9. Across the globe, people with intellectual disabilities, as well as racialized and minoritized populations, have been targeted by eugenics movements via forced sterilization (Bashford and Levine 2010; HRW 2011; Lira 2021).

10. Umm Lina never clarified what she meant by "the center," but I assumed she was referencing one of the many social or humanitarian-oriented civil society organizations that focus on children's rights, women's rights, and "awareness raising."

11. Kafer identifies a similar pattern in the case of Ashley X, writing that "the doctors involved in the case, Ashley's parents and supporters all draw on rhetoric and ideas nourished and developed from within disability rights movements, but to far different effects" (2013, 62).

12. In a study by Alyahya et al. (2019), 14.78 percent of their sample of 548 married women reported using implants and injectable hormonal contraceptives, while 6.2 percent reported using sterilization (158). Provider bias against injectables, which can also reduce or eliminate periods, is well-documented in Jordan (El-Khoury et al. 2015).

13. Studies have reported "partial gonadal dysfunction" in men with Down syndrome, but documented low fertility rates may also reflect social barriers to sexual activity (Parizot et al. 2019). Women with Down syndrome are fertile, although they typically go through early menopause, and approximately one in three women with Down syndrome will give birth to a child with Down syndrome (Parizot et al. 2019).

14. Ifta' is a verbal noun that literally means "the issuance of fatwas" rather than referring to either a singular fatwa or plural (*fatawa*).

15. It is possible to "search" for a fatwa that suits one's desired response (Agrama 2010), but people nevertheless tend to respect their authority.

16. A legal expert, Dr. Alazzeh is also Jordan's first blind member of Parliament and Jordan's current representative on the U.N. Committee on the Rights of Persons with Disabilities.

17. Jordan's 2017 *Shadow Report* reported that six hysterectomies were performed at a hospital in southern Jordan in 2015, but the authors also raised concerns about underreporting.

18. *Lihunna* (for them) marks the feminine plural in Arabic.

19. The question of masturbation never surfaced in reference to women's desire to find a boyfriend or husband. My own positionality, however, as neither kin nor a close intimate, as neither a wife nor a mother, certainly influenced whether women would broach this topic with me. Talk about menstruation was relatively banal; talk about sex was another matter entirely.

20. As previously noted, a premature or medically unnecessary hysterectomy creates a variety of health risks, and activists are currently trying to increase awareness of these dangers.

21. For a discussion of how these stereotypes operate in the context of the United States, see Block (2000).

CHAPTER 6   AGING UNCERTAINTIES

Portions of chapter 6 were previously published in Sargent (2021, 116–128).

1. Writing about transformations in middle-class childrearing in contemporary China, for example, Teresa Kuan examines how a confluence of political, cultural, and economic factors informed her interlocutors "sense that raising a child from birth to adulthood is fraught with uncertainty" (2015, 157).

2. Drawing on fieldwork in Vietnam, Tine Gammeltoft (2008) offers a compelling contrast during her intense exchange with Hoan, the father of a twenty-one-year-old man with physical disabilities. Despite his wife's pleas not to, Hoan openly shared his severe doubts about whether his other children or their spouses would care for their son. He described their futures as full of misery and fear, in "a shocking breach of the idealized picture of themselves that families usually present to outsiders" (578).

3. As documented by ethnographers of gender and labor in Jordan, not to mention substantial policy-focused literature, the limited entry of Jordanian women into the formal labor force stands in stark contrast to their extremely high rates of education. In urban areas, many middle- and upper-class women cycle through the formal labor market based on the demands and needs of their households. Working-class and poorer women find fewer and less accessible opportunities to work despite having a greater need for income.

4. In their work on "American disability worlds" (2024, 1), Faye Ginsburg and Rayna Rapp describe the "social production of moxie" as a process by which "parents move from isolation, becoming by necessity persistent, vigilant advocates for their children's diverse pedagogical needs" (83). They use moxie to account for the wide-ranging interventions and forms of resistance that parents cultivate, which may nevertheless remain outside more formal or traditional domains of political activism.

5. Approaching care as generative, explains the anthropologist Elana Buch, opens up "analytic possibilities for recognizing the transformative as well as reproductive potential of those inevitable moments of friction that occur amidst the messy day-to-day of making life happen" (2018, 18).

6. Congregate care settings are equally if not more stigmatized for older adults than for the disabled. Both cultural and religious traditions situate elder care as a child's duty and form of repayment to one's parents (Hammad et al. 2022). As converging forces—longer lifespans, shrinking family sizes, and migration abroad for education and work—undermine the sustainability of kinship-based home care, the question of elder care is particularly morally charged.

7. Jordan's Law No. 20 does not mirror the CRPD completely, but I have chosen to include portions of text from the latter. Notably, the provisions of the CRPD's Article 23 ("Respect for Home and the Family") are largely absent from Law No. 20. The provisions of the CRPD's Article 19 are addressed in Article 27 of Law No. 20. The law's overarching, binding principles of nondiscrimination and equality create several points of conflict with the formulations of legal capacity and consent articulated elsewhere in Jordanian legal canon (Ghaly 2019). Responding to questions from the CRPD committee about the Personal Status Act of 2010, which requires judicial authorization for persons with psychosocial and intellectual disabilities to marry, Jordan's CRPD committee expressed cautious optimism about their ongoing discussions with the Ministry of Religious Endowments, Islamic Affairs and Holy Places (CRPD 2017). But they reminded the CRPD committee that the latter retains jurisdiction over the Personal Status Law and all matters pertaining to it. This creates divergent interpretations of "legal capacity" and "equal recognition before the law."

8. Clause C of the CRPD's Article 19 states that "community services and facilities for the general population are available on an equal basis to persons with disabilities and are responsive

to their needs." I have omitted it from the section's epigraph given its broad purview and less direct bearing on the ethnographic data.

9. The term *markez* directly translates to "center" rather than "institution." Most of my interlocutors referred to residential institutions as "centers" (*marakez*) because many of these organizations' names included this term. In legal and policy briefs, residential institutions are referred to using the phrases *dar al-iwa'* (shelter, literally, "a house of accommodation") or *dar al-r'iaya al-iwa'iyya* (house of residential care). See note 14 for more on the definition of an institution.

10. Many semantic overlaps exist between *dar* and bayt, both in Jordan and other Arabic-speaking countries.

11. Anthropological literature on houses and housing is central to the discipline and spans a variety of theoretical approaches (Samanani and Lenhard 2019).

12. As Mariam Ababsa explains, "The patriarchal hierarchy can be considered as much a marker of the Christian communities as it is of the Muslim communities. . . . Christians apply Shari'a law to matters of inheritance, as there is no clause within the canon laws of the eleven Christian churches of Jordan concerning the distribution of shares" (2017, 113).

13. Geoffrey Hughes suggests that, at least in some cases, this decision may reflect a strategic calculation that enables women to "trade their share in return for a sort of moral claim on their male relatives" (2022, 371; see also Moors 1995).

14. The label "institution" refers to "long-stay residential facilities that *segregate and confine* people with disabilities" (Open Society Foundation 2019; my emphasis). By design, institutions "deprive residents of essential freedoms, segregate them from their communities, suppress individual choice and personal expression, and foster a perception that people with disabilities are different and unable to take a place in society" (Open Society Foundation 2019). They can be public or private, large or small; what institutions share are cultural norms and explicit policies of hierarchy, surveillance, and separation.

15. "Home" is mentioned four other times in the CRPD. In the first two cases (preamble and Article 16), "home" appears as part of the phrase "within and outside the home." Article 22, "Respect for Privacy," asserts that persons with disability have the right to be free from "arbitrary or unlawful interference with his or her privacy, family, home or correspondence." Article 23, "Respect for Home and the Family," discusses the right to marry, the right to access family-planning services, and the right to retain fertility, but the text of the clauses does not reference home.

16. Elizabeth Davis's (2012) ethnography of psychiatric deinstitutionalization in Thrace remains a notable exception to the focus on deinstitutionalization in Global North contexts. Anthropologists and historians of the Southwest Asia and North Africa (SWANA) region have begun to excavate *histories* and contemporary forms of institutionalization in Lebanon and the broader Levant (Abi-Rached 2020; Moghnieh 2022; Tsacoyianis 2021). These accounts do not always engage with paradigms of disability, which perhaps reflects the more limited reach of disability models into the otherwise robust regional field of critical studies of psychiatry (Behrouzan 2016; Pandolfo 2018; Vinea 2018, 2023). While mental illness and disability are not synonymous, they are linked through shared histories of institutionalization and overlapping movements for deinstitutionalization.

17. Vanier was a devout Roman Catholic, and L'arche reflected and informed his theological commitments (McKearney 2017). Today, L'arche's website describes its mission as "invit[ing] people with and without intellectual disabilities to build community together" (2024). It remains "rooted in Christian gospel" but is "shaped by people of different beliefs, practices and religions." While L'arche programs continue to thrive, the organization has grappled with recent revelations that its revered founder sexually abused at least twenty-five nondisabled women in France through his involvement with a "hidden sect [that] that

identified people seeking spiritual guidance and exploited them for sexual purposes"
(Banerjee 2023).

18. These angels are known as the Kiraman Katibin, or honorable scribes/recorders, who
witness and document every good and bad deed. The accounts they record will be presented
on the Day of Judgment.

19. Nonaccountability generated value and vulnerability. Not having an account meant that
family members and caretakers became more accountable on that person's behalf, which
some used to justify the surveillance and restrictions they imposed on their kin, especially
beyond childhood (see chapter 5).

20. In his typological study of "benefit granting" in Islam, Kazuo Ohtsuka (1988) notes that
while Qur'anic references to *thawab* definitively refers to rewards granted in the afterlife, *'ajr*
ostensibly covers both rewards in this life or the afterlife. In everyday conversation, people
connected *'ajr* with the motivation of entering heaven. Anthropologists have elsewhere
described *'ajr* as a "religious merit" (Jansen 2004), "divine reward" (Deeb 2006, 149), or
"points with God" (Deeb 2006, 233) that facilitate entry to heaven.

21. Clause C refers to the right to retain fertility, which I have omitted from this section's
epigraph but explore extensively in chapter 5. Notably, and despite mirroring the CRPD in
many ways, Jordan's Law No. 20 does not explicitly address the right to marry, start a family, or
retain fertility.

22. This court-ordered stipulation connects to the issues discussed in note 3 about legal
capacity and marriage under Jordan's Personal Status Law.

23. While class and citizenship engendered massive differences between Umm Farid's and
Umm Sami's lifestyles, they were close in age. It is possible that their stance also reflected a
shared generational perspective, although many younger mothers of younger children
expressed similar opinions on the unsuitability of marriage.

24. Article 27, item 1, includes eleven separate clauses (a–k) that lay out principles of nondiscrimination, protection, and reasonable accommodation. Given the extensiveness of this list,
I have only included the opening text.

25. It was not clear to me whether they considered typical banter among colleagues as in and
of itself inappropriate.

26. Umm Sami literally used the adjective "normal" here, but I have translated it as "nondisabled" in the context of our conversation. For many of my interlocutors, "normal" communicated many possible meanings; it did not necessarily convey the pathologizing and
stigmatizing connotations criticized elsewhere by medical anthropologists and disability
studies scholars (Sargent 2025).

CHAPTER 7   ACCEPTANCE

1. Examples might include Ángela Covadonga Bachiller, who became Spain's first city coun-
cillor with Down syndrome in 2013, or Mar Galcerán, Spain's first parliamentarian with Down
syndrome in 2024. In a different vein of representation, Puerto Rico's Sofía Jirau became Victoria's Secret's first model with Down syndrome in 2022. In 2024, an ad featuring Madison
Tevlin, a model with Down syndrome, went viral on World Down Syndrome Day with its
powerful message about how stereotypes about Down syndrome become reality for people
with the condition. See the ad at https://www.youtube.com/watch?v=9HpLhxMFJR8&t=5s.

2. While not yet a reality, current and future gene-editing technologies might be applied to
the genomes of people with Down syndrome in pursuit of "improvement" or even "cure."
Fictional works like Daniel Keyes's classic short story *Flowers for Algernon* (1959) attest to the
presence of this cultural script.

3. I do not invoke "dwelling" in quite the same way as Tim Ingold, who has used the term in his extensive oeuvre. But I appreciate his point that "the trouble with 'dwelling' is that it sounds altogether too cosy and comfortable, conjuring up a haven of rest where all tensions are resolved . . . while we may acknowledge that dwelling is a way of being at home in the world, home is not necessarily a comfortable or pleasant place to be, nor are we alone there" (2005, 503).

4. The closure of special education centers was extraordinarily difficult for families and children. At the behest of families and activists, centers reopened far earlier than schools, albeit with special operating procedures (Weldali 2020).

5. Entire families have been eradicated from Gaza's civil registry over the past twenty-one months, as Israel wages a genocidal campaign against inhabitants of the besieged territory. This violence has intensified the stakes of kinship futures by highlighting their preciousness and their vulnerability.

REFERENCES

Ababneh, Sara. 2018. "'Do You Know Who Governs Us? The Damned Monetary Fund.'" Middle East Research and Information Project. June 30. https://merip.org/2018/06/do -you-know-who-governs-us-the-damned-monetary-fund/.

Ababsa, Myriam. 2013a. "The Amman Ruseifa-Zarqa Built-Up Area: The Heart of the National Economy." In *Atlas of Jordan: History, Territories and Society*, edited by Myriam Ababsa. Presses de l'Ifpo. https://doi.org/10.4000/books.ifpo.5044.

———. 2013b. "Changes in the Regional Distribution of the Population." In *Atlas of Jordan: History, Territories and Society*, edited by Myriam Ababsa. Presses de l'Ifpo. https://doi.org /10.4000/books.ifpo.5021.

———. 2013c. "The Socio-Economic Composition of the Population." In *Atlas of Jordan: History, Territories and Society*, edited by Myriam Ababsa. Presses de l'Ifpo. https://doi.org/10 .4000/books.ifpo.5021.

———. 2017. "The Exclusion of Women from Property in Jordan." *Hawwa: Journal of Women of the Middle East and the Islamic World* 15:107–128. https://doi.org/10.1163/15692086 -12341317.

Abbas, Saba. 2015. "'My Veil Makes Me Beautiful': Paradoxes of *Zeena* and Concealment in Amman." *Journal of Middle East Women's Studies* 11 (2): 139–160. https://doi.org/10.1215 /15525864-2886514.

Abdo, Nour, Nadia Ibraheem, Nail Obeidat, Ashley Graboski-Bauer, Anwar Batieha, Nada Altamimi, and Moawia Khatatbih. 2018. "Knowledge, Attitudes, and Practices of Women Toward Prenatal Genetic Testing." *Epigenetics Insights* 11 (December): 1–20. https://doi .org/10.1177/2516865718813122.

Abi-Rached, Joelle. 2020. ʿAṣfūriyyeh: A History of Madness, Modernity, and War in the Middle East. MIT Press.

Abu-Habib, Lina. 1997. *Gender and Disability: Women's Experiences in the Middle East*. Humanities Press.

Abu-Lughod, Lila. 1985. "Honor and the Sentiments of Loss in a Bedouin Society." *American Ethnologist* 12 (2): 245–261. https://doi.org/10.1525/ae.1985.12.2.02a00040.

———. 1986. *Veiled Sentiments: Honor and Poetry in a Bedouin Society*. University of California Press.

———, ed. 1998. *Remaking Women: Feminism and Modernity in the Middle East*. Princeton University Press.

Abu Moghli, Mira, Émilie MacIsaac, and Emily Wiseman. 2018. "Transporting Jordanian Women into Employment." Policy paper on National Issues from a Gender Perspective. USAID Takamol. In the author's possession.

Achilli, Luigi. 2014. "Disengagement from Politics: Nationalism, Political Identity, and the Everyday in a Palestinian Refugee Camp in Jordan." *Critique of Anthropology* 34 (2): 234–257. https://doi.org/10.1177/0308275X13519276.

———. 2015. "Al-Wihdat Refugee Camp: Between Inclusion and Exclusion." *Jadaliyya* (blog). February 12, 2015. https://www.jadaliyya.com/Details/31776.

Açiksöz, Salih Can. 2019. *Sacrificial Limbs: Masculinity, Disability, and Political Violence in Turkey*. University of California Press.

Adely, Fida J. 2009. "Educating Women for Development: The Arab Human Development Report 2005 and the Problem with Women's Choices." *International Journal of Middle East Studies* 41 (1): 105–122. https://doi.org/10.1017/S0020743808090144.

———. 2012a. *Gendered Paradoxes: Educating Jordanian Women in Nation, Faith, and Progress.* University of Chicago Press. http://ebookcentral.proquest.com/lib/cudenver/detail.action?docID=990882.

———. 2012b. "'God Made Beautiful Things': Proper Faith and Religious Authority in a Jordanian High School." *American Ethnologist* 39 (2): 297–312. https://doi.org/10.1111/j.1548-1425.2012.01365.x.

———. 2016. "A Different Kind of Love: Compatibility (Insijam) and Marriage in Jordan." *Arab Studies Journal* 24 (2): 102–127. https://www.jstor.org/stable/44742882.

———. 2024. *Working Women in Jordan: Education, Migration, and Aspiration.* University of Chicago Press.

Agarwal, Ashwin, Lauren C. Sayres, Mildred K. Cho, Robert Cook-Deegan, and Subhashini Chandrasekharan. 2013. "Commercial Landscape of Noninvasive Prenatal Testing in the United States: Commercialization of Noninvasive Prenatal Testing." *Prenatal Diagnosis* 33 (6): 521–531. https://doi.org/10.1002/pd.4101.

Agrama, Hussein Ali. 2010. "Ethics, Tradition, Authority: Toward an Anthropology of the Fatwa." *American Ethnologist* 37 (1): 2–18. https://doi.org/10.1111/j.1548-1425.2010.01238.x.

Ahmed, Leila. 1992. *Women and Gender in Islam: Historical Roots of a Modern Debate.* Reissue ed. Yale University Press.

Akrami, Musa. 2017. "From Logic in Islam to Islamic Logic." *Logica Universalis* 11 (1): 61–83. https://doi.org/10.1007/s11787-017-0158-3.

Alazeh, Muhannad, and Civil Society Coalition. 2012. "'Mirror of Reality and Tool for Change': Civil Society Report on the Status of Implementation of the Convention on the Rights of Persons with Disabilities in Jordan." In the author's possession.

Alazzeh, Muhannad. n.d. "قل ولا تقل في مجال حقوق الأشخاص ذوي الإعاق." https://hcd.gov.jo/ebv4.0/root_storage /ar /eb _list _page /%D8%AF%D9%84%D9%8A%D9%84 _%D9%82%D9%84 _%D9%88%D9%84%D8%A7 _%D8%AA%D9%82%D9%84_.pdf.

AlBawaba. 2012. "بالفيديو:خلف جدران الصمت..جريمة تشعل الشارع الأردني." May 17. https://www.albawaba.com/ar.

Alhalaseh, Lana J. 2019. "Population Ageing in the Eastern Mediterranean Countries: A Regional Overview of the Situation Jordan." *Middle East Journal of Age and Ageing* 16 (1): 36–54. https://doi.org/10.5742/MEJAA.2019.93622.

Al Khatib, Jamal, and Fareed Al Khatib. 2008. "Educating Students with Mild Intellectual Disabilities in Regular Schools in Jordan." *Journal of the International Association of Special Education* 9:109–116. https://jamalalkhateeb.com/abhath/Educating%20students%20with%20intellectual%20disabilities.pdf.

Allan, Diana, ed. 2021. *Voices of the Nakba: A Living History of Palestine.* Pluto Press.

Almala, Afaf. 2014. "Gender and Guardianship in Jordan: Femininity, Compliance, and Resistance." PhD diss., SOAS, University of London. https://eprints.soas.ac.uk/view/people/Almala=3AAfaf=3A=3A.html.

Almasarweh, Issa S. 2003. "Adolescent and Youth Reproductive Health in Jordan." Policy Project, USAID. https://pdf.usaid.gov/pdf_docs/Pnact791.pdf.

Al-Mohammad, Hayder. 2010. "Towards an Ethics of Being-With: Intertwinements of Life in Post-Invasion Basra." *Ethnos* 75 (4): 425–446. https://doi.org/10.1080/00141844.2010.544394.

Al-Nakib, Mai. 2014. "'The People Are Missing': Palestinians in Kuwait." *Deleuze Studies* 8 (1): 23–44. https://doi.org/10.3366/dls.2014.0132.

Alodat, Ali, Hisham Almakanin, and Marshall Zumberg. 2014. "Inclusive Education Within the Jordanian Legal Framework: Overview of Reality and Suggestions for Future." *International Journal of Academic Research in Business and Social Sciences* 4 (5). https://doi.org/10.6007/IJARBSS/v4-i5/850.

Alon, Yoav. 2009. *The Making of Jordan: Tribes, Colonialism and the Modern State*. I. B. Tauris.

Aloul, Sahar, Randa Naffa, and May Mansour. 2018. "Gender in Public Transportation: A Perspective of Women Users of Public Transportation." Friedrich Ebert Siftung & Sadaqa. https://www.fes-jordan.org/publications/publications-from-jordan/?tx_digbib_digbibpublicationlist.

Al-Wedyan, Ashraf Bader Alddin, and Alia Mohammed Al-Oweidi. 2021. "The Effectiveness of Portage Early Intervention Program in Improving Adaptive Behavior Skills with Intellectual Disorders." *International Education Studies* 15 (1): 16. https://doi.org/10.5539/ies.v15n1p16.

Alyahya, Mohammad S., Heba H. Hijazi, Hussam A. Alshraideh, Nihaya A. Al-sheyab, Dana Alomari, Sara Malkawi, Sarah Qassas, Samah Darabseh and Yousef S. Khader. 2019. "Do Modern Family Planning Methods Impact Women's Quality of Life? Jordanian Women's Perspectives." *Health and Quality of Life Outcomes* (17): 154–170. https://doi.org/10.1186/s12955-019-1226-6.

Amawi, Abla. 2000. "Gender and Citizenship in Jordan." In *Gender and Citizenship in the Middle East*, edited by Suad Joseph. Syracuse University Press.

Amman Net. 2007. "لحمايتهن من الاغتصاب،عائلات تستئصل أرحام بناتها." May 26. https://ammannet.net.

———. 2012. "خلف جدران الصمت: فيلم يكشف بكاميرا سرية عن إساءة لأطفال معوقين بالأردن." May 13. https://ammannet.net.

Amnesty International. 2019. "Imprisoned Women, Stolen Children: Policing Sex, Marriage, and Pregnancy in Jordan." https://www.amnesty.org/en/documents/mde16/0831/2019/en/.

Amr, Muna. 2011. "Teacher Education for Inclusive Education in the Arab World: The Case of Jordan." *PROSPECTS* 41 (3): 399–413. https://doi.org/10.1007/s11125-011-9203-9.

Annamma, Subini Ancy. 2018. *The Pedagogy of Pathologization: Dis/Abled Girls of Color in the School-Prison Nexus*. Routledge.

Antonarakis, Stylianos E., Brian G. Skotko, Michael S. Rafii, Andre Strydom, Sarah E. Pape, Diana W. Bianchi, Stephanie L. Sherman, and Roger H. Reeves. 2020. "Down Syndrome." *Nature Reviews Disease Primers* 6 (1): 1–20. https://doi.org/10.1038/s41572-019-0143-7.

Arabiat, Diana H., N. M. Alqaissi, and A. M. Hamdan-Mansour. 2011. "Children's Knowledge of Cancer Diagnosis and Treatment: Jordanian Mothers' Perceptions and Satisfaction with the Process." *International Nursing Review* 58 (4): 443–449. https://doi.org/10.1111/j.1466-7657.2011.00899.x.

Artiles, Alfredo, Elizabeth B. Kozleski, and Federico R. Waitoller, eds. 2011. *Inclusive Education: Examining Equity on Five Continents*. Harvard Education Press.

Assaad, Ragui, Caroline Krafft, and Dominique J. Rolando. 2017. "The Role of Housing Markers in the Timing of Marriage in Egypt, Jordan, and Tunisia." Working Paper No. 1081. Economic Research Forum, March 18–20, Amman, Jordan. https://ideas.repec.org/p/erg/wpaper/1081.html#:~:text=We%20find%20that%20Egypt's%20rental,inadequate%20supply%20of%20rental%20housing.

Atia, Mona. 2013. *Building a House in Heaven: Pious Neoliberalism and Islamic Charity in Egypt*. University of Minnesota Press.

Aulino, Felicity. 2017. "Narrating the Future: Population Aging and the Demographic Imaginary in Thailand." *Medical Anthropology* 36 (4): 319–331. https://doi.org/10.1080/01459740.2017.1287181.

———. 2019. *Rituals of Care: Karmic Politics in an Aging Thailand.* Cornell University Press.

Awamleh, Zaid, and Kamel Dorai. 2023. "The Spatial Governance of the Syrian Refugee Crisis in Jordan: Refugees Between Urban Settlements and Encampment Policies." *CMI Report* 2023:3. https://www.cmi.no/publications/8909-the-spatial-governance-of-the-syrian-refugee-crisis-in-jordan.

Bagenstos, Samuel R. 2014. "The Disability Cliff." *Democracy Journal.* December 8. https://democracyjournal.org/magazine/35/the-disability-cliff/.

Banerjee, Sidhartha. 2023. "Report Finds That L'Arche Co-Founder Jean Vanier Sexually Abused 25 Women." *CBC.* January 31. https://www.cbc.ca/news/canada/montreal/jean-vanier-sexual-abuse-women-1.6731500.

Barakat, R., Lisa Drylie, and Jennifer Nash. 2004. "The Portage Project: An Overview of a Model for Early Childhood Education." https://faculty.unlv.edu/jgelfer/ECE707/ThePortageProject%28GROUP%29.doc

Bashford, Alison, and Philippa Levine, eds. 2010. *The Oxford Handbook of the History of Eugenics.* Oxford University Press.

Battles, Heather T., and Lenore Manderson. 2008. "The Ashley Treatment: Furthering the Anthropology of/on Disability." *Medical Anthropology* 27 (3): 219–226. https://doi.org/10.1080/01459740802222690.

Baylouny, Anne Marie. 2006. "Creating Kin: New Family Associations as Welfare Providers in Liberalizing Jordan." *International Journal of Middle East Studies* 38:349–368. https://doi.org/10.1017/S0020743806383018.

———. 2008. "Militarizing Welfare: Neo-Liberalism and Jordanian Policy." *Middle East Journal* 62 (2): 277–303. http://www.jstor.org/stable/25482510.

———. 2010. *Privatizing Welfare in the Middle East: Kin Mutual Aid Associations in Jordan and Lebanon.* Indiana University Press.

Bazna, Maysaa S., and Tarek A. Hatab. 2005. "Disability in the Qur'an: The Islamic Alternative to Defining, Viewing, and Relating to Disability." *Journal of Religion, Disability & Health* 9 (1): 5–27. https://doi.org/10.1300/J095v09n01_02.

BBC Arabic. 2012. "خلف جدران الصمت." *BBC News* عربي. May 14. https://www.bbc.com/arabic/tvandradio/2012/05/120514_xtracarehomes.

Beaudevin, Claire. 2013. "Old Diseases and Contemporary Crisis: Inherited Blood Disorders in the Sultanate of Oman." *Anthropology & Medicine* 20 (2): 175–189. https://doi.org/10.1080/13648470.2013.805317.

Behrouzan, Orkideh. 2016. *Prozak Diaries: Psychiatry and Generational Memory in Iran.* Stanford University Press.

Ben-Moshe, Liat, Chris Chapman, and Alison C. Carey, eds. 2014. *Disability Incarcerated: Imprisonment and Disability in the United States and Canada.* Palgrave Macmillan.

Benson, Sarah K. 2020. "The Evolution of Jordanian Inclusive Education Policy and Practice." *FIRE: Forum for International Research in Education* 6 (1). https://doi.org/10.32865/fire202061177.

Bérubé, Michael. 2018. "Don't Let My Son Plunge off the 'Disability Cliff' When I'm Gone." *USA Today*, April 2. https://www.usatoday.com/story/opinion/2018/04/02/dont-let-my-son-plunge-off-disability-cliff-column/443138002/.

Betran, Ana Pilar, Jiangfeng Ye, Ann-Beth Moller, João Paulo Souza, and Jun Zhang. 2021. "Trends and Projections of Caesarean Section Rates: Global and Regional Estimates." *BMJ Global Health* 6 (6). https://doi.org/10.1136/bmjgh-2021-005671.

Biehl, João, and Peter Locke. 2017. "Ethnographic Sensorium." In *Unfinished: The Anthropology of Becoming*, edited by João Biehl and Peter Locke. Duke University Press.

Biehl, João, and Federico Neiburg. 2021. "Oikography: Ethnographies of House-ing in Critical Times." *Cultural Anthropology* 36 (4): 539–547. https://doi.org/10.14506/ca36.4.01.

Bishara, Amahl. 2023. "Decolonizing Middle East Anthropology." *American Ethnologist* 50 (3): 396–408. https://doi.org/10.1111/amet.13200.

Bittles, Alan H. 2005. "Endogamy, Consanguinity and Community Disease Profiles." *Community Genetics* 8 (1): 17–20. https://doi.org/ 10.1159/000083332.

Bittles, Alan H., and E. J. Glasson. 2004. "Clinical, Social, and Ethical Implications of Changing Life Expectancy in Down Syndrome." *Developmental Medicine & Child Neurology* 46 (4). https://doi.org/10.1017/S0012162204000441.

Block, Ellen, and Will Mcgrath. 2019. *Infected Kin: Orphan Care and AIDS in Lesotho*. Rutgers University Press. https://doi.org/10.2307/j.ctvscxrqh.

Block, Pamela. 2000. "Sexuality, Fertility, and Danger: Twentieth-Century Images of Women with Cognitive Disabilities." *Sexuality and Disability* 18 (4): 239–254. https://doi-org.aurarialibrary.idm.oclc.org/10.1023/A:1005642226413.

———. 2007. "Institutional Utopias, Eugenics, and Intellectual Disability in Brazil." *History and Anthropology* 18 (2): 177–196. https://doi.org/10.1080/02757200701702851.

———. 2020. "Activism, Anthropology, and Disability Studies in Times of Austerity: In Collaboration with Sini Diallo." *Current Anthropology* 61 (S21): S68–S75. https://doi.org/10.1086/705762.

Blum, Linda M. 2015. *Raising Generation Rx: Mothering Kids with Invisible Disabilities in an Age of Inequality*. New York University Press.

Bourdieu, Pierre. 1977. *Outline of a Theory of Practice*. Translated by Richard Nice. Cambridge University Press.

Brue, Alan W., and Thomas Oakland. 2001. "The Portage Guide to Early Intervention: An Evaluation of Published Evidence." *School Psychology International* 22 (3): 243–252. https://doi.org/10.1177/0143034301223001.

Buch, Elana D. 2015. "Anthropology of Aging and Care." *Annual Review of Anthropology* 44 (1): 277-293. http://www.annualreviews.org/doi/10.1146/annurev-anthro-102214-014254.

———. 2018. Z. New York University Press.

Buchbinder, Mara. 2015. *All in Your Head: Making Sense of Pediatric Pain*. University of California Press.

Bull, Marilyn J., Tracy Trotter, Stephanie L. Santoro, Celanie Christensen, Randall W. Grout, and the Council on Genetics. 2022. "Health Supervision for Children and Adolescents with Down Syndrome." *Pediatrics* 149 (5): e2022057010. https://doi.org/10.1542/peds.2022-057010.

Cameron, David Lansing. 2021. "Efficacy of the Portage Early Intervention Programme 'Growing: Birth to Three' for Children Born Prematurely." *Early Child Development and Care* 191 (16): 2558–2569. https://doi.org/10.1080/03004430.2020.1723571.

Carey, Allison C., Richard K. Scotch, and Pamela Block. 2020. *Allies and Obstacles: Disability Activism and Parents of Children with Disabilities*. Temple University Press.

Carlson, Licia, and Eva Feder Kittay. 2010. "Introduction: Rethinking Philosophical Presumptions in Light of Cognitive Disability." In *Cognitive Disability and Its Challenge to Moral Philosophy*, edited by Eva Feder Kittay and Licia Carlson. Wiley.

Carr, Janet, and Suzanne Collins. 2018. "50 Years with Down Syndrome: A Longitudinal Study." *Journal of Applied Research in Intellectual Disabilities* 31 (5): 743–750. https://doi.org/10.1111/jar.12438.

Carsten, Janet. 2000. "Introduction: Cultures of Relatedness." In *Cultures of Relatedness: New Approaches to the Study of Kinship*. Cambridge University Press. https://ctools.umich.edu /access/content/group/9514a145-ea39-4722-9797-68e1e8945d43/REQUIRED%20 READINGS/Carsten%202000%20Intro%20-%20Cultures%20of%20Relatedness.pdf.

Cascio, M. Ariel, and Eric Racine, eds. 2019. *Research Involving Participants with Cognitive Disability and Difference: Ethics, Autonomy, Inclusion, and Innovation*. Oxford University Press.

Centers for Disease Control and Prevention, National Center for Health Statistics. 2024a. "Births—Method of Delivery." April 9. https://www.cdc.gov/nchs/fastats/delivery.htm.

———. 2024b. "Disability Impacts All of Us." https://www.cdc.gov/ncbddd/disabilityand health/infographic-disability-impacts-all.html.

CESA5 (Cooperative Educational Service Agency 5). 2023. "Cooperative Educational Service Agency 5." https://www.cesa5.org/.

Chen, Mel Y. 2016. "'The Stuff of Slow Constitution': Reading Down Syndrome for Race, Disability, and the Timing That Makes Them So." *Somatechnics* 6 (2): 235–248. https://doi .org/10.3366/soma.2016.0193.

———. 2023. *Intoxicated: Race, Disability, and Chemical Intimacy Across Empire*. Duke University Press.

Cipriani, Gabriele, Sabrina Danti, Cecilia Carlesi, and Mario Di Fiorino. 2018. "Aging with Down Syndrome: The Dual Diagnosis: Alzheimer's Disease and Down Syndrome." *American Journal of Alzheimer's Disease & Other Dementias* 33 (4): 253–262. https://doi.org /10.1177/1533317518761093.

Clarke, Adele E., Janet K. Shim, Laura Mamo, Jennifer Ruth Fosket, and Jennifer R. Fishman. 2003. "Biomedicalization: Technoscientific Transformations of Health, Illness, and U.S. Biomedicine." *American Sociological Review* 68 (2): 161–194. https://doi.org/10.2307 /1519765.

Clarke, Morgan. 2007. "Closeness in the Age of Mechanical Reproduction: Debating Kinship and Biomedicine in Lebanon and the Middle East." *Anthropological Quarterly* 80 (2): 379–402. https://doi.org/10.1353/anq.2007.0022.

———. 2009. *Islam and New Kinship: Reproductive Technology and the Shariah in Lebanon*. Berghahn Books.

Clift, Ashley Kieran, Carol A. C. Coupland, Ruth H. Keogh, Harry Hemingway, and Julia Hippisley-Cox. 2021. "COVID-19 Mortality Risk in Down Syndrome: Results from a Cohort Study of 8 Million Adults." *Annals of Internal Medicine* 174 (4): 572–576. https:// doi.org/10.7326/M20-4986.

Coombe, Rosemary J. 1990. "Barren Ground: Re-Conceiving Honour and Shame in the Field of Mediterranean Ethnography." *Anthropologica* 32 (2): 221–238.

Corker, Mairian. 2001. "Sensing Disability." *Hypatia* 16 (4): 34–52. https://doi.org/10.1111 /j.1527-2001.2001.tb00752.x.

CRPD (Convention on the Rights of Persons with Disabilities). 2017. "Response of the Hashemite Kingdom of Jordan to the List of Issues Sent by the Committee on the Rights of Persons with Disabilities." January 10. https://tbinternet.ohchr.org/_layouts/15/treaty bodyexternal/Download.aspx?symbolno=CRPD%2FC%2FJOR%2FQ%2F1%2FAdd .1&Lang=en.

Dabash, Rasha, and Farzaneh Roudi-Fahimi. 2008. "Abortion in the Middle East and North Africa." Population Reference Bureau. https://gynuity.org/assets/resources/polbrf_menaa bortion_en.pdf.

Dalal, Ayham. 2020. "The Refugee Camp as Site of Multiple Encounters and Realizations." *Review of Middle East Studies* 54 (2): 215–233. https://doi.org/10.1017/rms.2021.10.

Dar Al-Ifta'. 2009. "حكم إزالة رحم فتاة معاقة عقليًا." December 13. http://aliftaa.jo/fatwa/390.

———. 2014. "حرمة إزالة أرحام الفتيات ذوات الإعاقة (194) قرار." March 16. http://aliftaa.jo/decision/243.

———. 2015 "1993 2015." مسائل في الحمل والولادة. قرار رقم: (35). http://aliftaa.jo/decision/36.

Dasoqi, K. Al, R. Zeilani, M. Abdalrahim, and C. Evans. 2013. "Screening for Breast Cancer Among Young Jordanian Women: Ambiguity and Apprehension." *International Nursing Review* 60 (3): 351–357. https://doi.org/10.1111/inr.12025.

Davis, Elizabeth Anne. 2012. *Bad Souls: Madness and Responsibility in Modern Greece*. Duke University Press.

Deeb, Lara. 2006. *An Enchanted Modern: Gender and Public Piety in Shi'i Lebanon*. Princeton University Press.

Deeb, Lara, and Mona Harb. 2013. *Leisurely Islam: Negotiating Geography and Morality in Shi'ite South Beirut*. Princeton University Press.

Demeyere, Bruno. 2022. "Interview with His Royal Highness Prince Mired Bin Raad Zeid Al-Hussein of Jordan." *International Review of the Red Cross*, no. 922 (November). http://international-review.icrc.org/articles/interview-with-his-royal-highness-prince-mired-bin-raad-zeid-al-hussein-of-jordan-922.

Department of Social Affairs UAE. 2025. "أصحاب الهمم (الأشخاص ذوي الإعاقة)." https://u.ae/ar-ae/information-and-services/social-affairs/people-of-determination.

Dewachi, Omar. 2015. "When Wounds Travel." *Medicine Anthropology Theory* 2 (3): 61. https://doi.org/10.17157/mat.2.3.182.

Dey, Arpita, Krishnendu Bhowmik, Arpita Chatterjee, Swagata Sinha, and Kanchan Mukhopadhyay. 2013. "Down Syndrome Related Muscle Hypotonia: Association with COL6A3 Functional SNP Rs2270669." *Frontiers in Genetics* 4 (April). https://doi.org/10.3389/fgene.2013.00057.

Dokumacı, Arseli. 2023. *Activist Affordances: How Disabled People Improvise More Habitable Worlds*. Duke University Press.

Dolmage, Jay. 2017. *Academic Ableism: Disability and Higher Education*. University of Michigan Press.

Dols, Michael. 1992. *Majnun: The Madman in Medieval Islamic Society*. Oxford University Press.

DOS (Department of Statistics) [Jordan]. 2015. "General Population and Housing Census 2015."

———. 2021. "The Reality of Disability." http://www.dos.gov.jo/dos_home_e/main/population/census2015/Disability%202021.pdf.

DOS (Department of Statistics) [Jordan] and ICF. 2019. *Jordan Population and Family Health Survey 2017–18*. http://dosweb.dos.gov.jo/products/dhs2017-2018/.

———. 2023. *Jordan Population and Family Health Survey 2023*. https://dhsprogram.com/pubs/pdf/FR388/FR388.pdf.

Douglas, Mary. 2002. *Purity and Danger: An Analysis of Concepts of Pollution and Taboo*. Routledge.

Down, John Langdon. 1866. "Observations on an Ethnic Classification of Idiots." *London Hospital Clinical Report* 3:259–262. https://www.nature.com/articles/hdy196669.

Dunn, Dana S., and Erin E. Andrews. 2015. "Person-First and Identity-First Language: Developing Psychologists' Cultural Competence Using Disability Language." *American Psychologist* 70 (3): 255–264. https://doi.org/10.1037/a0038636.

Ehrenreich, Barbara, and Arlie Russell Hochschild, eds. 2004. *Global Woman: Nannies, Maids, and Sex Workers in the New Economy*. 1st ed. Holt Paperbacks.

Eli-Long, Rebecca, and Hannah Quinn. 2022. "Rupturing 'Capacity to Consent': Toward Anti-Ableist Research Relations." *Cultural Anthropology: Theorizing the Contemporary*.

https://culanth.org/fieldsights/rupturing-capacity-to-consent-toward-anti-ableist
-research-relations.

El-Khoury, Marianne, Rebecca Thornton, Minki Chatterji, and Soon Kyu Choi. 2015. "Effectiveness of Evidence-Based Medicine on Knowledge, Attitudes, and Practices of Family
Planning Providers: A Randomized Experiment in Jordan." *BMC Health Services Research*
15 (1). https://doi.org/10.1186/s12913-015-1101-z.

El-Mohammad, Abdallah. 2019. "Syria: Mentally Challenged Girls Undergo Forced Hysterectomies for Fear of Rape and Menstruation—Daraj." November 14. https://daraj.media
/en/syria-mentally-challenged-girls-undergo-forced-hysterectomy-for-fear-of-rape-and
-menstruation/.

El-Seedi, Hesham R., Shaden A. M. Khalifa, Nermeen Yosri, Alfi Khatib, Lei Chen, Aamer Saeed,
Thomas Efferth, and Rob Verpoorte. 2019. "Plants Mentioned in the Islamic Scriptures (Holy
Qur'ān and Ahadith): Traditional Uses and Medicinal Importance in Contemporary Times."
Journal of Ethnopharmacology 243 (October): 112007. https://doi.org/10.1016/j.jep.2019.112007.

El Shakry, Omnia. 1998. "Schooled Mothers and Structured Play: Child Rearing in Turn-of-the-
Century Egypt." In *Remaking Women*, edited by Lila Abu-Lughod. Feminism and Modernity in the Middle East. Princeton University Press. https://doi.org/10.2307/j.ctt7sck7.9.

———. 2011. "Youth as Peril and Promise: The Emergence of Adolescent Psychology in Postwar Egypt." *International Journal of Middle East Studies* 43 (4): 591–610. https://doi.org
/10.1017/S002074381100119X.

Elyachar, Julia. 2011. "The Political Economy of Movement and Gesture in Cairo: Movement
and Gesture in Cairo." *Journal of the Royal Anthropological Institute* 17 (1): 82–99. https://
doi.org/10.1111/j.1467-9655.2010.01670.x.

El Zein, Rayya. 2020. "Toward a Dialectic of Discrepant Cosmopolitanisms." *Middle East Journal
of Culture and Communication* 13 (2): 170–189. https://doi.org/10.1163/18739865-01302007.

Engelke, Dörthe. 2019. "Jordan." In *Filiation and the Protection of Parentless Children: Towards a
Social Definition of the Family in Muslim Jurisdictions*, edited by Nadjma Yassari, Lena-
Maria Möller, and Marie-Claude Najm. T.M.C. Asser Press.

Erevelles, Nirmala. 2011. *Disability and Difference in Global Contexts: Enabling a Transformative
Body Politic*. Palgrave Macmillan.

ESCWA (United Nations Economic and Social Commission for Western Asia). 2018a. *Disability in the Arab Region 2018*. https://www.unescwa.org/publications/disability-arab
-region-2018.

———. 2018b. *Jordan: Gender, Justice, and the Law*. https://www.unescwa.org/sites/default
/files/event/materials/jordan-adjusted.pdf.

Espinosa, Joaquin M. 2020. "Down Syndrome and COVID-19: A Perfect Storm?" *Cell Reports
Medicine* 1 (2): 100019. https://doi.org/10.1016/j.xcrm.2020.100019.

Esson, James. 2013. "A Body and a Dream at a Vital Conjuncture: Ghanaian Youth, Uncertainty and the Allure of Football." *Geoforum* 47:84–92. https://doi.org/10.1016/j.geoforum
.2013.03.011.

Estreich, George. 2016. "An Open Letter to Medical Students: Down Syndrome, Paradox, and
Medicine." *AMA Journal of Ethics* 18 (4): 438–441. https://doi.org/10.1001/journalofethics
.2016.18.4.mnar1-1604.

Evans, Ruth. 2014. "Parental Death as a Vital Conjuncture? Intergenerational Care and
Responsibility Following Bereavement in Senegal." *Social & Cultural Geography* 15 (5):
547–570. https://doi.org/10.1080/14649365.2014.908234.

Faour, Basma, Youssef Hajjar, Ghanem Bibi, Maysoun Chehab, and Rima Zaazaa. 2006.
"Comparative, Regional Analysis of ECCE in Four Arab Countries (Lebanon, Jordan,
Syria, and Sudan)." Working paper for the *Education for All Global Monitoring Report 2007*,

Strong Foundations: Early Childhood Care and Education, UNESCO. https://unesdoc
.unesco.org/ark:/48223/pf0000147440.

Farahat, Hind, and Kritsin E. Cheney. 2015. "A Facade of Democracy: Negotiating the Rights
of Orphans in Jordan." *Global Studies of Childhood* 5 (2): 146–157. https://doi.org/10.1177
/2043610615586101.

Feldman, Ilana. 2017. "Humanitarian Care at the Ends of Life." *Cultural Anthropology* 32 (1):
42–67. https://doi.org/10.14506/ca32.1.06.

———. 2018. *Life Lived in Relief: Humanitarian Predicaments and Palestinian Refugee Politics.*
University of California Press.

FHI 360 and EPDC (Education Policy and Data Center). 2018. *Jordan National Education
Profile 2018 Update.* https://www.epdc.org/sites/default/files/documents/EPDC_NEP
_2018_Jordan.pdf.

Fietz, Helena. 2020a. "Negotiating Care: Living Arrangements and Adults with Cognitive Disabilities in South Brazil." *Développement Humain, Handicap et Changement Social/Human
Development, Disability, and Social Change* 26 (1): 37–47. https://doi.org/10.7202/1068189ar.

———. 2020b. "The Paradox of Autonomy and Care for Mothers of Adults with Disabilities
in Brazil." *The CASTAC Blog.* http://blog.castac.org/2020/05/the-paradox-of-autonomy
-and-care-for-mothers-of-adults-with-disabilities-in-brazil/.

Fischbach, Michael R. 2000. *State, Society, and Land in Jordan.* Brill.

Flaskerud, Jacquelyn H. 1988. "Is the Likert Scale Format Culturally Biased?" *Nursing Research*
37 (3): 185.

Foley, Charlene, and Orla G. Killeen. 2019. "Musculoskeletal Anomalies in Children with Down
Syndrome: An Observational Study." *Archives of Disease in Childhood* 104 (5): 482–487.
https://doi.org/10.1136/archdischild-2018-315751.

Fost, Norman. 2020. "'The Hopkins Mongol Case': The Dawn of the Bioethics Movement."
Pediatrics 146 (S1): S3–S8. https://doi.org/10.1542/peds.2020-0818C.

Foucault, Michel. 1980. *Power/Knowledge: Selected Interviews and Other Writings, 1972–1977.*
Edited by Colin Gordon. Translated by Colin Gordon, Leo Marshall, John Mepham, and
Kate Soper. Pantheon Books.

Frantz, Elizabeth. 2008. "Of Maids and Madams." *Critical Asian Studies* 40 (4): 609–638.
https://doi.org/10.1080/14672710802505323.

———. 2010. "Buddhism by Other Means: Sacred Sites and Ritual Practice Among Sri
Lankan Domestic Workers in Jordan." *Asia Pacific Journal of Anthropology* 11 (3–4): 268–292.
https://doi.org/10.1080/14442213.2010.511629.

———. 2013. "Jordan's Unfree Workforce: State-Sponsored Bonded Labour in the Arab
Region." *Journal of Development Studies* 49 (8): 1072–1087. https://doi.org/10.1080/0022
0388.2013.780042.

Friedner, Michele Ilana. 2015. *Valuing Deaf Worlds in Urban India.* Rutgers University Press.

———. 2019. "Praying for Rights: Cultivating Deaf Worldings in Urban India." *Anthropological
Quarterly* 92 (2): 403–426. https://doi.org/10.1353/anq.2019.0020.

———. 2020. "Disability, Anonymous Love, and Interworldly Socials in Urban India." *Current
Anthropology* 61 (S21): S37–S45. https://doi.org/10.1086/704942.

———. 2022a. "From Hoping to Expecting: Cochlear Implantation and Habilitation in
India." *Cultural Anthropology* 37 (1): 125–149. https://doi.org/10.14506/ca37.1.10.

———. 2022b. *Sensory Futures: Cochlear Implants and Sensory Infrastructures in India.* University of Minnesota Press.

Friedner, Michele Ilana, and Tyler Zoanni. 2018. "Disability from the South: Toward a Lexicon."
Somatosphere (blog). December 17. http://somatosphere.net/2018/12/disability-from-the
-south-toward-a-lexicon.html.

Fullwiley, Duana. 2004. "Discriminate Biopower and Everyday Biopolitics: Views on Sickle Cell Testing in Dakar." *Medical Anthropology* 23 (2): 157–194. https://doi.org/10.1080/01459740490448939.

Fung, Heidi. 1999. "Becoming a Moral Child: The Socialization of Shame Among Young Chinese Children." *Ethos* 27 (2): 180–209. https://doi.org/10.1525/eth.1999.27.2.180.

Gabbay, Shaul M. 2014. "The Status of Palestinians in Jordan and the Anomaly of Holding a Jordanian Passport." *Journal of Political Sciences & Public Affairs* 2 (1). https://doi.org/10.4172/2332-0761.1000113.

Gabiam, Nell. 2012. "When 'Humanitarianism' Becomes 'Development': The Politics of International Aid in Syria's Palestinian Refugee Camps." *American Anthropologist* 114 (1): 95–107. https://doi.org/10.1111/j.1548-1433.2011.01399.x.

———. 2016. *The Politics of Suffering: Syria's Palestinian Refugee Camps.* Indiana University Press.

Gammeltoft, Tine M. 2008. "Childhood Disability and Parental Moral Responsibility in Northern Vietnam: Towards Ethnographies of Intercorporeality." *Journal of the Royal Anthropological Institute* 14 (4): 825–842. https://doi.org/10.1111/j.1467-9655.2008.00533.x.

———. 2014a. *Haunting Images: A Cultural Account of Selective Reproduction in Vietnam.* University of California Press.

———. 2014b. "Toward an Anthropology of the Imaginary: Specters of Disability in Vietnam." *Ethos* 42 (2): 153–174. https://doi.org/10.1111/etho.12046.

Gausman, Jewel, Areej Othman, Iqbal Lutfi Hamad, Maysoon Dabobe, Insaf Daas, and Ana Langer. 2019. "How Do Jordanian and Syrian Youth Living in Jordan Envision Their Sexual and Reproductive Health Needs? A Concept Mapping Study Protocol." *BMJ Open* 9:e027266. https://doi.org/10.1136/bmjopen-2018-027266.

Gebel, Michael, and Stefanie Heyne. 2016. "Delayed Transitions in Times of Increasing Uncertainty: School-to-Work Transition and the Delay of First Marriage in Jordan." *Research in Social Stratification and Mobility* 46 (December): 61–72. https://doi.org/10.1016/j.rssm.2016.01.005.

Gennep, Arnold van. 1961. *The Rites of Passage.* University of Chicago Press.

Gernsbacher, Morton Ann. 2017. "Editorial Perspective: The Use of Person-First Language in Scholarly Writing May Accentuate Stigma." *Journal of Child Psychology and Psychiatry* 58 (7): 859–861. https://doi.org/10.1111/jcpp.12706.

Ghaly, Mohammed M. 2008. "Physical and Spiritual Treatment of Disability in Islam: Perspectives of Early and Modern Jurists." *Journal of Religion, Disability & Health* 12 (2): 105–143. https://doi.org/10.1080/15228960802160647.

———. 2016. "Disability in the Islamic Tradition." *Religion Compass* 10 (6): 149–162. https://doi.org/10.1111/rec3.12202.

———. 2019. "The Convention on the Rights of Persons with Disabilities and the Islamic Tradition: The Question of Legal Capacity in Focus." *Journal of Disability & Religion* 23 (3): 251–278. https://doi.org/10.1080/23312521.2019.1613943.

Ghannam, Farha. 2011. "Mobility, Liminality, and Embodiment in Urban Egypt." *American Ethnologist* 38 (4): 790–800. https://doi.org/10.1111/j.1548-1425.2011.01337.x.

———. 2013. *Live and Die like a Man: Gender Dynamics in Urban Egypt.* Stanford University Press.

Giacaman, Rita. 2023. "The Limitations of Deinstitutionalization: The Case of the Israeli-Occupied Palestinian West Bank." *Journal of Palestine Studies* 52 (4): 76–86. https://doi.org/10.1080/0377919X.2023.2285635.

Ginsburg, Faye, and Rayna Rapp. 2013. "Disability Worlds." *Annual Review of Anthropology* 42 (1): 53–68. https://doi.org/10.1146/annurev-anthro-092412-155502.

———. 2024. *Disability Worlds*. Duke University Press.

Glasson, E. J., S. G. Sullivan, R. Hussain, B. A. Petterson, P. D. Montgomery, and A. H. Bittles. 2002. "The Changing Survival Profile of People with Down's Syndrome: Implications for Genetic Counselling." *Clinical Genetics* 62 (5): 390–393. https://doi.org/10.1034/j.1399-0004.2002.620506.x.

Glenn, Evelyn Nakano. 2010. *Forced to Care: Coercion and Caregiving in America*. Harvard University Press.

Good, Mary-Jo Delvecchio. 2007. "The Medical Imaginary and the Biotechnical Embrace: Subjective Experiences of Clinical Scientists and Patients." In *Subjectivity: Ethnographic Investigations*, edited by João Biehl, Byron Good, and Arthur Kleinman. University of California Press.

Goodley, Dan. 2013. "Dis/Entangling Critical Disability Studies." *Disability & Society* 28 (5): 631–644. https://doi.org/10.1080/09687599.2012.717884.

Goodley, Dan, Bill Hughes, and Lennard Davis, eds. 2012. *Disability and Social Theory*. Palgrave Macmillan UK. https://doi.org/10.1057/9781137023001.

Gordon, Jennifer. 2020. "The Obstacles to Decent Work for Migrants in Jordan: A Discussion with Alia Hindawi." *Civil Society Review* June. https://doi.org/10.28943/CSR.004.003.

Grech, Shaun. 2012. "Disability and the Majority World: A Neocolonial Approach." In *Disability and Social Theory: New Developments and Directions*, edited by Dan Goodley, Bill Hughes, and Lennard Davis. Palgrave Macmillan. https://doi.org/10.1057/9781137023001.

Grech, Shaun, and Karen Soldatic, eds. 2016. *Disability in the Global South: The Critical Handbook*. Springer.

Guardian Staff. 2024. "US Intelligence Casts Doubt on Israeli Claims of UNRWA-Hamas Links, Report Says." *Guardian*, February 22. https://www.theguardian.com/world/2024/feb/22/us-intelligence-unrwa-hamas.

Hacking, Ian. 1999. *The Social Construction of What?* Harvard University Press.

———. 2004. "Between Michel Foucault and Erving Goffman: Between Discourse in the Abstract and Face-to-Face Interaction." *Economy and Society* 33 (3): 277–302. https://doi.org/10.1080/0308514042000225671.

Hadidi, Muna S., and Jamal M. Al Khateeb. 2015. "Special Education in Arab Countries: Current Challenges." *International Journal of Disability, Development and Education* 62 (5): 518–530. https://doi.org/10.1080/1034912X.2015.1049127.

Hall, Sarah Marie. 2022. "Reproduction, Life-Course and Vital Conjunctures in the Context of Austerity." *Medical Anthropology: Cross Cultural Studies in Health and Illness* 41 (6–7): 732–746. https://doi.org/10.1080/01459740.2021.1951261.

Hamamy, Hanan, Stylianos E. Antonarakis, Luigi Luca Cavalli-Sforza, Samia Temtamy, Giovanni Romeo, Leo P. Ten Kate, Robin L. Bennett, et al. 2011. "Consanguineous Marriages, Pearls and Perils: Geneva International Consanguinity Workshop Report." *Genetics in Medicine* 13 (9): 841–847. https://doi.org/10.1097/GIM.0b013e318217477f.

Hamamy, Hanan, L. Jamhawi, J. Al-Darawsheh, and K. Ajlouni. 2005. "Consanguineous Marriages in Jordan: Why Is the Rate Changing with Time?" *Clinical Genetics* 67 (6): 511–516. https://doi.org/10.1111/j.1399-0004.2005.00426.x.

Hamdy, Sherine F. 2008. "When the State and Your Kidneys Fail: Political Etiologies in an Egyptian Dialysis Ward." *American Ethnologist* 35 (4): 553–569. https://doi.org/10.1111/j.1548-1425.2008.00098.x.

———. 2012. *Our Bodies Belong to God: Organ Transplants, Islam, and the Struggle for Human Dignity in Egypt*. University of California Press.

Hammad, Suzanne H., Suhad Daher-Nashif, Tanya Kane, and Noor Al-Wattary. 2022. "Sociocultural Insights on Dementia Care-Giving in Arab and Muslim Communities: The Perspectives of Family Care-Givers." *Ageing & Society* (2022): 1–28. https://doi.org/10.1017/S0144686X22000277.

Hanafi, Sari, Leila Hilal, and Lex Takkenberg, eds. 2014. *UNRWA and Palestinian Refugees: From Relief and Works to Human Development*. Routledge.

Hartblay, Cassandra. 2017. "Good Ramps, Bad Ramps: Centralized Design Standards and Disability Access in Urban Russian Infrastructure." *American Ethnologist* 44 (1): 9–22. https://doi.org/10.1111/amet.12422.

Hashim, Mohammad. 2024. "Developmental Stages: An Islamic Psychology Perspective." *Journal of Spirituality and Mental Health*, 1–24. Online ahead of print. https://doi.org/10.1080/19349637.2024.2439438.

Hasso, Frances. 2011. *Consuming Desires: Family Crisis and the State in the Middle East*. Stanford University Press.

Hauswedell, Charlotte. 2013. "Jordan: Journalist Uncovers Widespread Child Abuse." *DW Akademie* (blog). October 14, 2013. https://akademie.dw.com/en/jordan-journalist-uncovers-widespread-child-abuse/a-17156018.

HCD (Higher Council for the Rights of Persons with Disabilities). 2019. "الإعاقة بالأشخاص ذوي الإعاقة." الإستراتيجية الوطنية لبدائل دور الإيواء الحكومية والخاصة." https://www.mosd.gov.jo.

HCD (Higher Council for the Rights of Persons with Disabilities) and Bana Center. 2016. "واقع خدمات وبرامج التدخل المبكر في المملكة الأردنية الهاشمية للفئات من عمر سنتين إلى خمس سنوات" https://hcd.gov.jo.

Herrera, Linda, and Asef Bayat. 2010. *Being Young and Muslim: New Cultural Politics in the Global South and North*. Oxford University Press.

Herzfeld, Michael. 1980. "Honour and Shame: Problems in the Comparative Analysis of Moral Systems." *Man* 15 (2): 339. https://doi.org/10.2307/2801675.

Hessini, Leila. 2007. "Abortion and Islam: Policies and Practice in the Middle East and North Africa." *Reproductive Health Matters* 15 (29): 75–84. https://www.jstor.org/stable/25475294.

Hoodfar, Homa. 1997. *Between Marriage and the Market: Intimate Politics and Survival in Cairo*. University of California Press.

Hourani, Najib B. 2014. "Urbanism and Neoliberal Order: The Development and Redevelopment of Amman." *Journal of Urban Affairs* 36 (S2): 634–649. https://doi.org/10.1111/juaf.12092.

Hourani, Najib B., and Ahmed Kanna. 2014. "Neoliberal Urbanism and the Arab Uprisings: A View from Amman." *Journal of Urban Affairs* 36 (S2): 650–662. https://doi.org/10.1111/juaf.12136.

Howard-Jones, Norman. 1979. "On the Diagnostic Term 'Down's Disease.'" *Medical History* 23 (1): 102–104. https://doi.org/10.1017/S0025727300051048.

Howell, Signe. 2003. "Kinning: Creating Life-Trajectories in Adoptive Families." *Journal of the Royal Anthropological Institute* 9 (3): 465–484. https://www.jstor.org/stable/3134598.

———. 2006. *The Kinning of Foreigners: Transnational Adoption in a Global Perspective*. Berghahn Books.

HRW (Human Rights Watch). 2010. *Stateless Again*. February 1. https://www.hrw.org/report/2010/02/01/stateless-again/palestinian-origin-jordanians-deprived-their-nationality.

———. 2011. "Sterilization of Women and Girls with Disabilities." November 10. https://www.hrw.org/news/2011/11/10/sterilization-women-and-girls-disabilities.

———. 2019. "Jordan: Insufficient Disability Rights Funding." *Human Rights Watch* (blog). December 23. https://www.hrw.org/news/2019/12/23/jordan-insufficient-disability-rights-funding.

———. 2020. *Living in Chains: Shackling of People with Psychosocial Disabilities Worldwide*. October 6. https://www.hrw.org/report/2020/10/06/living-chains/shackling-people-psychosocial-disabilities-worldwide.

———. 2023. *Trapped: How Male Guardianship Policies Restrict Women's Travel and Mobility in the Middle East and North Africa*. July 18. https://www.hrw.org/report/2023/07/18/trapped/how-male-guardianship-policies-restrict-womens-travel-and-mobility-middle.

———. 2024. "Gaza: US, UK Outliers in Holding Back UNRWA Funding." https://www.hrw.org/news/2024/07/18/gaza-us-uk-outliers-holding-back-unrwa-funding.

Hughes, Bill, and Kevin Paterson. 1997. "The Social Model of Disability and the Disappearing Body: Towards a Sociology of Impairment." *Disability & Society* 12 (3): 325–340. https://doi.org/10.1080/09687599727209.

Hughes, Geoffrey F. 2015. "Infrastructures of Legitimacy: The Political Lives of Marriage Contracts in Jordan: Infrastructures of Legitimacy." *American Ethnologist* 42 (2): 279–294. https://doi.org/10.1111/amet.12130.

———. 2016. "The Proliferation of Men: Markets, Property, and Seizure in Jordan." *Anthropological Quarterly* 89 (4): 1081–1108. https://doi.org/10.1353/anq.2016.0069.

———. 2017. "The Chastity Society: Disciplining Muslim men." *Journal of the Royal Anthropological Institute* 23 (2): 267–284. https://doi.org/10.1111/1467-9655.12606.

———. 2019. "Tribes Without Sheikhs? Technological Change, Media Liberalization, and Authority in Networked Jordan." Working Paper No. 24. Program on Governance and Local Development at Gothenburg, Gothenberg, Sweden. https://papers.ssrn.com/sol3/papers.cfm?abstract_id=3810578.

———. 2021. *Kinship, Islam, and the Politics of Marriage in Jordan: Affection and Mercy*. Indiana University Press.

———. 2022. "Engineering Gender, Engineering the Jordanian State: Beyond the Salvage Ethnography of Middle-Class Housewifery in the Middle East." *Critique of Anthropology* 42 (4): 359–380. https://doi.org/10.1177/0308275X221139151.

Humanity and Inclusion. 2022. "Disability-Inclusive Education in Jordan." https://www.hi.org/sn_uploads/document/IE_Jordan_Factsheet_April-2022_Final.pdf.

ICNL (International Center for Not-For-Profit Law). 2024. "Jordan." https://www.icnl.org/resources/civic-freedom-monitor/jordan.

Ingold, Tim. 2005. "Epilogue: Towards a Politics of Dwelling: Conservation and Society." *Conversation and Society* 3 (2): 501–508. https://www.jstor.org/stable/26396589.

Ingstad, Benedicte. 1995. "Mph aa Yadimo—a Gift from God: Perspectives on 'Attitudes' Towards Disabled Persons." In *Disability and Culture*, edited by Benedicte Ingstad and Susan Reynolds Whyte. University of California Press.

Inhorn, Marcia C. 1994. *Quest for Conception: Gender, Infertility and Egyptian Medical Traditions*. University of Pennsylvania Press.

———. 2003. *Local Babies, Global Science: Gender, Religion and In Vitro Fertilization in Egypt*. Routledge.

———. 2012. *The New Arab Man: Emergent Masculinities, Technologies, and Islam in the Middle East*. Princeton University Press.

———. 2015. *Cosmopolitan Conceptions: IVF Sojourns in Global Dubai*. Duke University Press.

Inhorn, Marcia C., and Soraya Tremayne. 2016. "Islam, Assisted Reproduction, and the Bioethical Aftermath." *Journal of Religion and Health* 55 (2): 422–430. https://doi.org/10.1007/s10943-015-0151-1.

IRCKHF (Information and Research Center–King Hussein Foundation). 2017. "Empowering Care Leavers in Jordan." March 7. https://haqqi.s3.eu-north-1.amazonaws.com/2018-01/IRCKHF_FHI360_ECLJ_V1_Eng.pdf.

Islam, M. Mazharul. 2021. "Consanguineous Marriage and Its Relevance to Divorce, Polygyny and Survival of Marriage: Evidence from a Population-Based Analysis in Jordan." *Annals of Human Biology* 48 (1): 30–36. https://doi.org/10.1080/03014460.2021.1877354.

Islam, M. Mazharul, Faisal M. Ababneh, and M. D. Hasinur Rahaman Khan. 2018. "Consanguineous Marriage in Jordan: An Update." *Journal of Biosocial Science* 50 (4): 573–578. https://doi.org/10.1017/S0021932017000372.

Ivry, Tsipy. 2006. "At the Back Stage of Prenatal Care: Japanese Ob-Gyns Negotiating Prenatal Diagnosis." *Medical Anthropology Quarterly* 20 (4): 441–468. https://doi.org/10.1525/maq.2006.20.4.441.

———. 2010. *Embodying Culture: Pregnancy in Japan and Israel*. Rutgers University Press.

Jabril, Reem. 2021. "إزالة أرحام ذوات الإعاقة. جرائم طبية بدوافع اجتماعية قاسية." *Noon Post*, December 10. https://www.noonpost.com/42603/.

Jackson, Aaron J. 2021. *Worlds of Care: The Emotional Lives of Fathers Caring for Children with Disabilities*. University of California Press.

Jackson, Michael. 2005. *Existential Anthropology: Events, Exigencies, and Effects*. 1st ed. Berghahn Books.

———. 2012. *Lifeworlds: Essays in Existential Anthropology*. University of Chicago Press.

Jacob, Wilson Chacko. 2011. *Working Out Egypt: Effendi Masculinity and Subject Formation in Colonial Modernity, 1870–1940*. Duke University Press.

Jansen, Willy. 1987. *Women Without Men: Gender and Marginality in an Algerian Town*. E. J. Brill.

———. 2004. "The Economy of Religious Merit: Women and Ajr in Algeria." *Journal of North African Studies* 9 (4): 1–17. https://doi.org/10.1080/1362938042000326263.

Jean-Klein, Iris. 2000. "Mothercraft, Statecraft, and Subjectivity in the Palestinian Intifada." *American Ethnologist* 27 (1): 100–127. http://www.jstor.org/stable/647128.

Jenkins, Janice H. 2010. "Psychopharmaceutical Self and Imaginary in the Social Field of Psychiatric Treatment." In *Pharmaceutical Self: The Global Shaping of Experience in an Age of Psychopharmacology*, edited by Janice H. Jenkins. SAR Press.

Jensehaugen, Jørgen. 2020. "Jordan and COVID-19: Effective Response at a High Cost." Middle East Policy Brief. Peace Research Institute. Accessed June 28, 2025. https://cdn.cloud.prio.org/files/49cdb1ee-aa52-490d-a23e-8b1cd00270b9.

Johnson-Hanks, Jennifer. 2002. "On the Limits of Life Stages in Ethnography: Toward a Theory of Vital Conjunctures." *American Anthropologist* 104 (3): 865–880. https://doi.org/10.1525/aa.2002.104.3.865.

Jordan Times. 2018. "13 Per Cent of Jordanian Households Spend More Than Jd20,000 a Year." November 14. https://jordantimes.com/news/local/13-cent-jordanian-households-spend-more-jd20000-year.

Joseph, Suad. 1993. "Gender and Relationality Among Arab Families in Lebanon." *Feminist Studies* 19 (3): 465–486. https://doi.org/10.2307/3178097.

Kafer, Alison. 2013. *Feminist, Queer, Crip*. Indiana University Press.

———. 2019. "Crip Kin, Manifesting." *Catalyst: Feminism, Theory, Technoscience* 5 (1): 1–37. https://doi.org/10.28968/cftt.v5i1.29618.

Kandiyoti, Deniz. 1988. "Bargaining with Patriarchy." *Gender and Society* 2 (3): 274–290. https://www.jstor.org/stable/190357.

———. 1991. *Women, Islam and the State*. Macmillan.

Kanter, Arlene S. 2007. "The Promise and Challenge of the United Nations Convention on the Rights of Persons with Disabilities." *Syracuse Journal of International Law and Commerce* 34 (2): 287–322. https://papers.ssrn.com/sol3/papers.cfm?abstract_id=2109836.

Kaposy, Chris. 2018. *Choosing Down Syndrome: Ethics and New Prenatal Testing Technologies*. MIT Press.

———. 2023. *The Beautiful Unwanted: Down Syndrome in Myth, Memoir, and Bioethics*. McGill-Queen's Press.

Kashani-Sabet, Firoozeh. 2006. "The Politics of Reproduction: Maternalism and Women's Hygiene in Iran, 1896–1941." *International Journal of Middle East Studies* 38 (1): 1–29. https://doi.org/10.1017/S002074380641223X.

Kasnitz, Devva. 2020. "The Politics of Disability Performativity: An Autoethnography." *Current Anthropology* 61 (S21): S16–S25. https://doi.org/10.1086/705782.

Katz, Kimberly. 1995. *Jordanian Jerusalem: Holy Places and National Spaces.* University of Florida Press.

Kaya, Laura Pearl. 2009. "Dating in a Sexually Segregated Society: Embodied Practices of Online Romance in Irbid, Jordan." *Anthropological Quarterly* 82 (1): 251–278. https://doi.org/10.1353/anq.0.0043.

———. 2010. "The Criterion of Consistency: Women's Self-Presentation at Yarmouk University, Jordan." *American Ethnologist* 37 (3): 526–538. https://doi.org/10.1111/j.1548-1425.2010.01270.x.

Keyes, Daniel. 1959. *Flowers for Algernon.* 1st ed. Harcourt.

Khader, Yousef S., Mohammad S. Alyahya, Nihaya A. Al-Sheyab, Khulood K. Shattnawi, Hind Rajeh Saqer, and Anwar Batieha. 2018. "Evaluation of Maternal and Newborn Health Services in Jordan." *Journal of Multidisciplinary Healthcare* 2018 (September 5): 439–456. https://doi.org/10.2147/JMDH.S171982.

Khalaf, Inaam A., Fathieh Abu-Moghli, Lynn Clark Callister, and Rowida Rasheed. 2008. "Jordanian Women's Experiences with the Use of Traditional Family Planning." *Health Care for Women International* 29 (5): 527–538. https://doi.org/10.1080/07399330801949632.

Khalidi, Rashid. 2020. *The Hundred Years' War on Palestine: A History of Settler Colonialism and Resistance, 1917–2017.* Metropolitan Books/Henry Holt.

Khalidi, Walid. 1997. "Revisiting the UNGA Partition Resolution." *Journal of Palestine Studies* 27 (1): 5–21. https://doi.org/10.2307/2537806.

Khoury, S. A., and D. Massad. 1992. "Consanguineous Marriage in Jordan." *American Journal of Medical Genetics* 43 (5): 769–775. https://doi.org/10.1002/ajmg.1320430502.

Kim, Eunjung. 2011. "'Heaven for Disabled People': Nationalism and International Human Rights Imagery." *Disability & Society* 26 (1): 93–106. https://doi.org/10.1080/09687599.2011.529670.

———. 2017. *Curative Violence: Rehabilitating Disability, Gender, and Sexuality in Modern Korea.* Duke University Press.

Kittay, Eva Feder. 2019. "Forever Small: The Strange Case of Ashley X." In *Learning from My Daughter: The Value and Care of Disabled Minds.* 1st ed. Oxford University Press. https://doi.org/10.1093/oso/9780190844608.001.0001.

Kleinman, Arthur. 1992. "Local Worlds of Suffering: An Interpersonal Focus for Ethnographies of Illness Experience." *Qualitative Health Research* 2 (2): 127–134. https://doi.org/10.1177/104973239200200202.

———. 1999. "Moral Experience and Ethical Reflection: Can Ethnography Reconcile Them? A Quandary for 'the New Bioethics.'" *Daedalus* 128 (4): 69–97. https://www.jstor.org/stable/20027589.

Krafft, Caroline, and Ragui Assaad. 2012. "Employment's Role in Enabling and Constraining Marriage in the Middle East and North Africa." Working Paper No. 1080. Economic Research Forum, Cairo. https://doi.org/10.1007/s13524-020-00932-1.

Kuan, Teresa. 2015. *Love's Uncertainty: The Politics and Ethics of Child Rearing in Contemporary China.* University of California Press.

Kuttab, Daoud. 2023. "Jordan's Churches Approve Law on Equal Inheritance for Christian Women." *Christianity Today,* May 31. https://www.christianitytoday.com/ct/2023/may-web-only/jordan-churches-inheritance-women-men-equality-draft-law.html.

Landsman, Gail H. 2009. *Reconstructing Motherhood and Disability in the Age of Perfect Babies: Lives of Mothers of Infants and Toddlers with Disabilities.* Routledge.

Layne, Linda L. 1994. *Home and Homeland: The Dialogics of Tribal and National Identities in Jordan.* Princeton University Press.

Lee, Jerry W., Patricia S. Jones, Yoshimitsu Mineyama, and Xinwei Esther Zhang. 2002. "Cultural Differences in Responses to a Likert Scale." *Research in Nursing & Health* 25 (4): 295–306. https://doi.org/10.1002/nur.10041.

Lenner, Katharina. 2020. "'Biting Our Tongues': Policy Legacies and Memories in the Making of the Syrian Refugee Response in Jordan." *Refugee Survey Quarterly* 39:273–298. https://academic.oup.com/rsq/article/39/3/273/5843510.

Leppert, Rebecca, and Katherine Schaeffer. 2023. "8 Facts About Americans with Disabilities." Pew Research Center. July 24. https://www.pewresearch.org/short-reads/2023/07/24/8-facts-about-americans-with-disabilities.

Lira, Natalie. 2021. *Laboratory of Deficiency: Sterilization and Confinement in California, 1900–1950s.* University of California Press.

Livingston, Julie. 2005. *Debility and the Moral Imagination in Botswana.* Indiana University Press.

———. 2008. "Disgust, Bodily Aesthetics, and the Ethic of Being Human in Botswana." *Africa* 78 (2): 288–307.

Loh, Timothy Y. 2022. "Language in Medical Worlds: Hearing Technology for Deaf Jordanian Children." *Medical Anthropology: Cross-Cultural Studies in Health and Illness* 41 (1): 107–119. https://doi.org/10.1080/01459740.2021.2015346.

Löwy, Ilana. 2017. *Imperfect Pregnancies: A History of Birth Defects and Prenatal Diagnosis.* Johns Hopkins University Press.

Lutz, Catherine, and Lila Abu-Lughod, eds. 1990. *Language and the Politics of Emotion.* Studies in Emotion and Social Interaction. Cambridge University Press.

Lutz, Catherine, and Geoffrey M. White. 1986. "The Anthropology of Emotions." *Annual Review of Anthropology* 15:405–436. https://www.jstor.org/stable/2155767.

Ma, Zhiying. 2020. "Biopolitical Paternalism and Its Maternal Supplements: Kinship Correlates of Community Mental Health Governance in China." *Cultural Anthropology* 35 (2): 290–316. https://doi.org/10.14506/ca35.2.09.

MacDougall, Susan. 2019. "Ugly Feelings of Greed: The Misuse of Friendship in Working Class Amman." *Cambridge Journal of Anthropology* 37 (2): 74–89. https://doi.org/10.3167/cja.2019.370206.

———. 2021. "Felt Unfreedom: Reflecting on Ethics and Gender in Jordan." *Ethnos* 86 (3): 510–529. https://doi.org/10.1080/00141844.2019.1668449.

Maffi, Irene. 2013. *Women, Health and the State in the Middle East: The Politics and Culture of Childbirth in Jordan.* Bloomsbury Academic.

Maffi, Irene, and Liv Tonnessen. 2019. "The Limits of the Law: Abortion in the Middle East and North Africa." *Health and Human Rights Journal* 21 (2): 1–6. https://www.cmi.no/publications/7022-the-limits-of-law-abortion-in-the-middle-east-and-northern-africa.

Mahadeen, Ebtihal. 2013. "Doctors and Sheikhs: 'Truths' in Virginity Discourse in Jordanian Media." *Journal of International Women's Studies* 14 (4): 16. http://vc.bridgew.edu/jiws/vol14/iss4/7.

Malle, Louise, Cynthia Gao, Nicole Bouvier, Bethany Percha, and Dusan Bogunovic. 2020. "COVID-19 Hospitalization Is More Frequent and Severe in Down Syndrome and Affects Patients a Decade Younger." medRxiv. https://doi.org/10.1101/2020.05.26.20112748.

Malle, Louise, Cynthia Gao, Chin Hur, Han Q. Truong, Nicole M. Bouvier, Bethany Percha, Xiao-Fei Kong, and Dusan Bogunovic. 2021. "Individuals with Down Syndrome Hospitalized with COVID-19 Have More Severe Disease." *Genetics in Medicine* 23 (3): 576–580. https://doi.org/10.1038/s41436-020-01004-w.

Manderson, Lenore, and Narelle Warren. 2016. "'Just One Thing After Another': Recursive Cascades and Chronic Conditions." *Medical Anthropology Quarterly* 30 (4): 479–497. https://doi.org/10.1111/maq.12277.

Marcus, George. 1995. "Ethnography in/of the World System: The Emergence of Multi-Sited Ethnography." *Annual Review of Anthropology* 24:95–117. https://doi.org/10.1146/annurev.an.24.100195.000523.

Martin, Emily. 2007. *Bipolar Expeditions: Mania and Depression in American Culture.* Princeton University Press.

Martínez, José Ciro. 2017. "Leavening Neoliberalization's Uneven Pathways: Bread, Governance and Political Rationalities in the Hashemite Kingdom of Jordan." *Mediterranean Politics* 22 (4): 464–483. https://doi.org/10.1080/13629395.2016.1241613.

———. 2022. *States of Subsistence: The Politics of Bread in Contemporary Jordan.* Stanford University Press.

Mason, Olivia. 2021. "A Political Geography of Walking in Jordan: Movement and Politics." *Political Geography* 88:102392. https://doi.org/10.1016/j.polgeo.2021.102392.

Mason, Victoria. 2009. "Revenge and Terror: The Destruction of the Palestinian Community in Kuwait." In *Contemporary State Terrorism.* Routledge.

Massad, Joseph. 2001. *Colonial Effects: The Making of National Identity in Jordan.* Columbia University Press.

Mattingly, Cheryl. 2014a. *Moral Laboratories.* University of California Press.

———. 2014b. "The Moral Perils of a Superstrong Black Mother." *Ethos* 42 (1): 119–138. https://doi.org/10.1111/etho.12042.

Mauldin, Laura. 2016. *Made to Hear: Cochlear Implants and Raising Deaf Children.* University of Minnesota Press.

McClellan, Kate. 2019. "Becoming Animal People: Empathy Pedagogies and the Contested Politics of Care in Jordanian Animal Welfare Work." *Anthropological Quarterly* 92 (3): 787–815. https://doi.org/10.1353/anq.2019.0043.

McGranahan, Carole. 2018. "Ethnography Beyond Method: The Importance of an Ethnographic Sensibility." *Sites: A Journal of Social Anthropology and Cultural Studies* 15 (1): 1–10. https://doi.org/10.11157/sites-id373.

McGuire, Anne. 2016. *War on Autism: On the Cultural Logic of Normative Violence.* University of Michigan Press.

McKearney, Patrick. 2017. "L'Arche, Learning Disability, and Domestic Citizenship: Dependent Political Belonging in a Contemporary British City." *City & Society* 29 (2): 260–280. https://doi.org/10.1111/ciso.12126.

———. 2020. "What Escapes Persuasion: Why Intellectual Disability Troubles 'Dependence' in Liberal Societies." *Medical Anthropology: Cross Cultural Studies of Health and Illness* 40 (2): 155–168. https://doi.org/10.1080/01459740.2020.1805741.

———. 2021. "The Limits of Knowing Other Minds: Intellectual Disability and the Challenge of Opacity." *Social Analysis* 65 (1): 1–22. https://doi.org/10.3167/sa.2020.650101.

McLaughlin-Alcock, Colin. 2020. "Cultivated Affects: The Artistic Politics of Landscape and Memory in Amman's Gardens." *Visual Anthropology Review* 36 (2): 275–295. https://doi.org/10.1111/var.12219.

McRuer, Robert. 2006. *Crip Theory: Cultural Signs of Queerness and Disability.* New York University Press.

Meadows, Tey. 2018. *Trans Kids: Being Gendered in the Twenty-First Century.* University of California Press.

Meekosha, Helen, and Karen Soldatic. 2011. "Human Rights and the Global South: The Case of Disability." *Third World Quarterly* 32 (8): 1383–1397. https://doi.org/10.1080/01436597.2011.614800.

Meinert, Lotte, and Lone Grøn. 2019. "'It Runs in the Family': Exploring Contagious Kinship Connections." *Ethnos* 85 (4): 581–594. https://doi.org/10.1080/00141844.2019.1640759.

Meneley, Anne. 1996. *Tournaments of Value: Sociability and Hierarchy in a Yemeni Town*. University of Toronto Press.

———. 2003. "Scared Sick or Silly?" *Social Analysis* 47 (2). https://doi.org/10.3167/015597703782352989.

Méouchy, Nadine, Norig Neveu, and Myriam Ababsa. 2013. "The Hashemites and the Creation of Transjordan." In *Atlas of Jordan*, edited by Myriam Ababsa. Presses de l'Ifpo. https://doi.org/10.4000/books.ifpo.5010.

Mernissi, Fatima. 1975. *Beyond the Veil: Male-Female Dynamics in a Modern Muslim Society*. John Wiley & Sons.

Minich, Julie Avril. 2016. "Enabling Whom? Critical Disability Studies Now." *Lateral: Journal of the Cultural Studies Association* 5 (1). https://csalateral.org/issue/5-1/forum-alt-humanities-critical-disability-studies-now-minich/.

Ministry of Education [Jordan]. 2013. "Education Reform for Knowledge Economy Project (ERfKE II)." https://www.7iber.com.

———. 2018. *Strategic Plan: 2018–2022*. https://moe.gov.jo/sites/default/files/esp_english_final.pdf.

Ministry of Health [Jordan]. 2008. *Public Health Law of 2008*. https://www.moh.gov.jo/EN/List/Laws.

Mir-Hosseini, Ziba. 2000. *Marriage on Trial: A Study of Islamic Family Law*. I. B. Tauris.

Mitchell, David T. 2015. *The Biopolitics of Disability: Neoliberalism, Ablenationalism, and Peripheral Embodiment*. University of Michigan Press.

Mittermaier, Amira. 2012. "Dreams from Elsewhere: Muslim Subjectivities Beyond the Trope of Self-Cultivation." *Journal of the Royal Anthropological Institute* 18 (2): 247–265. https://doi.org/10.1111/j.1467-9655.2012.01742.x.

———. 2014. "Beyond Compassion: Islamic Voluntarism in Egypt." *American Ethnologist* 41 (3): 518–531. https://doi.org/10.1111/amet.12092.

Moghnieh, Lamia. 2022. "The Broken Promise of Institutional Psychiatry: Sexuality, Women and Mental Illness in 1950s Lebanon." *Culture, Medicine, and Psychiatry* 47 (May): 82–98. https://doi.org/10.1007/s11013-022-09786-1.

Mol, Annemarie. 2002. *The Body Multiple: Ontology in Medical Practice*. Duke University Press.

Mont, Daniel. 2007. "Measuring Disability Prevalence." Discussion Paper No. 0706. Social Protection Series. World Bank.

Moors, Annelies. 1995. *Women, Property and Islam: Palestinian Experiences, 1920–1990*. Cambridge University Press.

Moscoso, Melania, and R. Lucas Platero. 2017. "Cripwashing: The Abortion Debates at the Crossroads of Gender and Disability in the Spanish Media." *Continuum* 31 (3): 470–481. https://doi.org/10.1080/10304312.2016.1275158.

Musawah. 2017. "Overview of Muslim Family Laws and Practices: Jordan." https://www.musawah.org/wp-content/uploads/2019/03/Jordan-Overview-Table.pdf.

Musmar, Aya. 2020. "Witnessing as a Feminist Spatial Practice: Encountering the Refugee Camp Beyond Recognition." PhD diss., University of Sheffield. https://etheses.whiterose.ac.uk/25927/.

Nakamura, Karen. 2013. *A Disability of the Soul: An Ethnography of Schizophrenia and Mental Illness in Contemporary Japan*. Cornell University Press.

Nanes, Stefanie. 2010. "Hashemitism, Jordanian National Identity, and the Abu Odeh Episode." *Arab Studies Journal* 18 (1): 162–195. https://www.jstor.org/stable/27934081.

Nasri, Alix. 2017. "Migrant Domestic and Garment Workers in Jordan: A Baseline Analysis of Trafficking in Persons and Related Laws and Policies." Fundamental Principles and Rights at Work Branch. ILO. https://www.ilo.org/wcmsp5/groups/public/—ed_norm/—declaration/documents/publication/wcms_554812.pdf.

Nasser-Eddin, Nof. 2019. "Reflections on Theorising Class in Arabic-Speaking Countries." *Kohl: A Journal for Body and Gender Research* 5 (2): 98–103. https://kohljournal.press/theorising-class.

Nasser El-Dine, Sandra. 2018. "Love, Materiality, and Masculinity in Jordan: 'Doing' Romance with Limited Resources." *Men and Masculinities* 21 (3): 423–442. https://doi.org/10.1177/1097184X17748174.

Newman, Jess. 2018. "'There Is a Big Question Mark': Managing Ambiguity in a Moroccan Maternity Ward." *Medical Anthropology Quarterly* 33 (3): 386-402. http://doi.org/10.1111/maq.12510.

Nguyen, Xuan Thuy. 2023. "Decolonial Disability Studies." In *Crip Authorship: Disability as Method*, edited by Mara Mills and Rebecca Sanchez. New York University Press.

Nichols, Michelle, and Tom Perry. 2024. "Israel Yet to Show Evidence UNRWA Staff Are Members of Terrorist Groups, Review Finds." Reuters, April 22. https://www.reuters.com/world/middle-east/review-says-unrwa-has-robust-neutrality-steps-issues-persist-2024-04-22/.

Nimri, Nadine. 2016. "Will Survivors of Rape Be Given the Right to Abortion?" Translated by Orion Wilcox. *7iber*, May 11. https://www.7iber.com/society/will-survivors-of-rape-be-given-the-right-to-abortion/.

———. 2019. "دعوات لتمكين ضحايا الاغتصاب من تخلص آمن وقانوني للحمل." *Al Ghad*, May 6. https://alghad.com.

Noestlinger, Nette, and Gabriela Baczynska. 2024. "No Evidence from Israel to Back UNRWA Accusations, Says EU Humanitarian Chief." Reuters, March 14. https://www.reuters.com/world/no-evidence-israel-back-unrwa-accusations-says-eu-humanitarian-chief-2024-03-14/.

Oakland, Thomas. 1997. "A Multi-Year Home-Based Program to Promote Development of Young Palestinian Children Who Exhibit Developmental Delays." *School Psychology International* 18 (1): 29–39. https://doi.org/10.1177/0143034397181003.

Odgaard, Marie Rask Bjerre. 2021. "Contagious Heartaches: Relational Selfhood and Queer Care in Amman, Jordan." *Contemporary Islam* 15 (2): 187–199. https://doi.org/10.1007/s11562-020-00456-w.

———. 2022. "Queering 'Ayb in the Urban Landscapes of Amman." In *New Perspectives on Moral Change: Anthropologists and Philosophers Engage with Transformations of Life Worlds*, edited by Cecilie Eriksen and Nora Hämäläinen. Berghahn Books.

Ohtsuka, Kazuo. 1988. "Toward a Typology of Benefit-Granting in Islam." *Orient* 24:141–152. https://doi.org/10.5356/orient1960.24.141.

Oliver, Mike. 1990. *The Politics of Disablement*. Red Globe Press.

Open Society Foundation. 2019. "What Is Deinstitutionalization?" May. https://www.opensocietyfoundations.org/explainers/what-deinstitutionalization.

Ossman, Susan. 2002. *Three Faces of Beauty: Casablanca, Paris, Cairo*. Duke University Press. https://doi.org/10.1215/9780822383635.

Othman, Areej, Jamila Abuidhail, Abeer Shaheen, Ana Langer, and Jewel Gausman. 2022. "Parents' Perspectives Towards Sexual and Reproductive Health and Rights Education Among Adolescents in Jordan: Content, Timing and Preferred Sources of Information." *Sex Education* 22 (5): 628–639. https://doi.org/10.1080/14681811.2021.1975671.

Othman, Areej, Abeer Shaheen, Maysoon Otoum, Mohannad Aldiqs, Iqbal Hamad, May-soon Dabobe, Ana Langer, and Jewel Gausman. 2020. "Parent-Child Communication About Sexual and Reproductive Health: Perspectives of Jordanian and Syrian Parents." *Sexual and Reproductive Health Matters* 28 (1): 313–323. https://doi.org/10.1080/26410397.2020.1758444.

Pandolfo, Stefania. 2018. *Knot of the Soul: Madness, Psychoanalysis, Islam.* University of Chicago Press.

Pappe, Ilan. 2007. *The Ethnic Cleansing of Palestine.* Oneworld.

Parizot, Estelle, Rodolphe Dard, Nathalie Janel, and François Vialard. 2019. "Down Syndrome and Infertility: What Support Should We Provide?" *Journal of Assisted Reproduction and Genetics* 36 (6): 1063–1067. https://doi.org/10.1007/s10815-019-01457-2.

Parker, Christopher. 2009. "Tunnel-Bypasses and Minarets of Capitalism: Amman as Neoliberal Assemblage." *Political Geography* 28 (2): 110–120. https://doi.org/10.1016/j.polgeo.2008.12.004.

Parreñas, Rhacel Salazar. 2000. "Migrant Filipina Domestic Workers and the International Division of Reproductive Labor." *Gender & Society* 14 (4): 560–580. https://doi.org/10.1177/089124300014004005.

———. 2001. *Servants of Globalization.* Stanford University Press.

———. 2012. "The Reproductive Labour of Migrant Workers." *Global Networks* 12 (2): 269–275. https://doi.org/10.1111/j.1471-0374.2012.00351.x.

Patterson, Stephanie, and Pamela Block. 2019. "Disability, Vulnerability, and the Capacity to Consent—Oxford Scholarship." In *Research Involving Participants with Cognitive Disability and Difference: Ethics, Autonomy, Inclusion, and Innovation,* edited by M. Ariel Cascio and Eric Racine. Oxford University Press. https://login.aurarialibrary.idm.oclc.org.

Pearson, Thomas. 2023. *An Ordinary Future: Margaret Mead, the Problem of Disability, and a Child Born Different.* University of California Press.

Peletz, Michael. 1994. "Neither Reasonable nor Responsible: Contrasting Representations of Masculinity in a Malay Society." *Cultural Anthropology* 19 (2): 135–178. https://www.jstor.org/stable/656238.

Pérez, Michael Vicente. 2018. "Materializing the Nation in Everyday Life: On Symbols and Objects in the Palestinian Refugee Diaspora." *Dialectical Anthropology* 42 (4): 409–427. https://doi.org/10.1007/s10624-018-9505-x.

———. 2021. "Living as Enduring: The Struggle for Life Against the Limits of Refuge Among Gaza Refugees in Jordan." In *Un-Settling Middle Eastern Refugees: Regimes of Exclusion and Inclusion in the Middle East, Europe, and North America,* edited by Marcia C. Inhorn and Lucia Volk. Berghahn Books.

———. 2024. "Living as Stateless Palestinians in Jordan." *Sapiens* (blog). March 7. https://www.sapiens.org/culture/palestinian-refugees-exile-displacement-jordan/.

Peristiany, J. G., ed. 1965. *Honour and Shame—the Values of Mediterranean Society.* 1st ed. Weidenfeld & Nicholson.

Phillips, Sarah D. 2010. *Disability and Mobile Citizenship in Postsocialist Ukraine.* Indiana University Press.

Piepmeier, Alison. 2012. "Saints, Sages, and Victims: Endorsement of and Resistance to Cultural Stereotypes in Memoirs by Parents of Children with Disabilities." *Disability Studies Quarterly* 32 (1). https://doi.org/10.18061/dsq.v32i1.3031.

———. 2021. *Unexpected: Parenting, Prenatal Testing, and Down Syndrome.* New York University Press.

Piepzna-Samarasinha, Leah Lakshmi. 2018. *Care Work: Dreaming Disability Justice.* Arsenal Pulp Press.

Price, Margaret. 2011. *Mad at School: Rhetorics of Mental Disability and Academic Life*. University of Michigan Press.

———. 2015. "The Bodymind Problem and the Possibilities of Pain." *Hypatia* 30 (1): 268–284. https://doi.org/10.1111/hypa.12127.

Puar, Jasbir K. 2014. *The Right to Maim: Debility, Capacity, Disability*. Duke University Press.

Puschmann, Paul, and Koen Matthijs. 2012. "The Janus Face of the Demographic Transition in the Arab World: The Decisive Role of Nuptiality." Working Paper WOG/HD/2012-4. Centrum voor Sociologisch Onderzoek.

Rabinow, Paul. 2005. "Artificiality and Enlightenment: From Sociobiology to Biosociality." In *Anthropologies of Modernity*, edited by Jonathan Xavier Inda. Blackwell. https://doi.org/10.1002/9780470775875.ch7.

Rapp, Rayna. 1999. *Testing Women, Testing the Fetus: The Social Impact of Amniocentesis in America*. Routledge.

Rapp, Rayna, and Faye Ginsburg. 2001. "Enabling Disability: Rewriting Kinship, Reimagining Citizenship." *Public Culture* 13 (3): 533–556. https://doi.org/10.1215/08992363-13-3-533.

Rebhun, L. A. 1994. "Swallowing Frogs: Anger and Illness in Northeast Brazil." *Medical Anthropology Quarterly*, n.s., 8 (4): 360–382.

Richardson, Kristina L. 2012. *Difference and Disability in the Medieval Islamic World: Blighted Bodies*. Edinburgh University Press.

Rispler-Chaim, Vardit. 2007. *Disability in Islamic Law*. Springer.

Roberts, Elizabeth F. S. 2008. "Biology, Sociality and Reproductive Modernity in Ecuadorian In-Vitro Fertilization: The Particulars of Place." In *Biosocialities, Genetics and the Social Sciences: Making Biologies and Identities*, edited by Sahra Gibbon and Carlos Novas. Routledge.

Rodríguez-Hernández, M. Luisa, and Eladio Montoya. 2011. "Fifty Years of Evolution of the Term Down's Syndrome." *Lancet* 378 (9789): 402. https://doi.org/10.1016/S0140-6736(11)61212-9.

Rubaii, Kali. 2020. "Birth Defects and the Toxic Legacy of War in Iraq." Middle East Research and Information Project, no. 296. October. https://merip.org/2020/10/birth-defects-and-the-toxic-legacy-of-war-in-iraq-296/.

Runswick-Cole, Katherine, and Sara Ryan. 2019. "Liminal Still? Unmothering Disabled Children." *Disability & Society* 34 (7–8): 1125–1139. https://doi.org/10.1080/09687599.2019.1602509.

Rutherford, Danilyn. 2020. "Proximity to Disability." *Anthropological Quarterly* 93 (1): 1453–1481. https://doi.org/10.1353/anq.2020.0018.

Rutherford, Kenneth R. 2007. "Jordan and Disability Rights: A Pioneering Leader in the Arab World." *Review of Disability Studies: An International Journal* 3 (4). https://www.rdsjournal.org.

Ryan, Curtis R. 2011. "Political Opposition and Reform Coalitions in Jordan." *British Journal of Middle Eastern Studies* 38 (3): 367–390. https://doi.org/10.1080/13530194.2011.621699.

Ryan, Curtis R., and Jillian Schwedler. 2004. "Return to Democratization or New Hybrid Regime? The 2003 Elections in Jordan." *Middle East Policy* 11 (2): 138–151. https://doi.org/10.1111/j.1061-1924.2004.00158.x.

Ryan, Sara, and Katherine Runswick-Cole. 2008. "Repositioning Mothers: Mothers, Disabled Children and Disability Studies." *Disability & Society* 23 (3): 199–210. https://doi.org/10.1080/09687590801953937.

Saleh, Zainab. 2020. *Return to Ruin: Iraqi Narratives of Exile and Nostalgia*. Stanford University Press.

Salem, Rania. 2012. "Trends and Differentials in Jordanian Marriage Behavior: Marriage Timing, Spousal Characteristics, Household Structure, and Matrimonial Expenditures." Working Paper 668. Economic Research Forum, Giza, Egypt. https://doi.org/10.1093/acprof: oso/9780198702054.003.0007.

Samanani, Farhan, and Johannes Lenhard. 2019. "House and Home." *The Open Encyclopedia of Anthropology*, December 9. Facsimile of the first edition in *The Cambridge Encyclopedia of Anthropology*. https://www.anthroencyclopedia.com/entry/house-and-home.

Samin, Nadav. 2015. *Of Sand or Soil*. Princeton University Press.

Sanal, Aslihan. 2011. *New Organs Within Us: Transplants and the Moral Economy*. Duke University Press.

Sargent, Christine. 2019. "Development." Somatosphere. April 1. https://somatosphere.com/2019/development.html/.

———. 2020. "The Stakes of (Not) Knowing." *Medicine Anthropology Theory* 7 (2): 10–32. https://doi.org/10.17157/mat.7.2.683.

———. 2021. "Kinship, Connective Care, and Disability in Jordan." *Medical Anthropology: Cross Cultural Studies in Health and Illness* 40 (2): 116–128. https://doi.org/10.1080/0145 9740.2020.1858295.

———. 2025. "Claiming Normal: Disability, Stigma, and Relationality in Amman." *Medical Anthropology Quarterly* e7003. http://doi.org/10.1111/maq.70003.

Sarouphim, Ketty M., and Sara Kassem. 2022. "Use of the Portage Curriculum to Impact Child and Parent Outcome in an Early Intervention Program in Lebanon." *Early Years* 42 (October): 528–542. https://www.tandfonline.com/doi/abs/10.1080/09575146.2020 .1818186.

Scalenghe, Sara. 2014. *Disability in the Ottoman Arab World: 1500–1800*. Cambridge University Press.

Schalk, Sami. 2018. *Bodyminds Reimagined: (Dis)Ability, Race, and Gender in Black Women's Speculative Fiction*. Duke University Press.

Scheper-Hughes, Nancy, and Margaret M. Lock. 1987. "The Mindful Body: A Prolegomenon to Future Work in Medical Anthropology." *Medical Anthropology Quarterly* 1 (1): 6–41. https://doi.org/10.1525/maq.1987.1.1.02a00020.

Schielke, Samuli. 2008. "Boredom and Despair in Rural Egypt." *Contemporary Islam* 2 (3): 251–270. https://doi.org/10.1007/s11562-008-0065-8.

———. 2009. "Being Good in Ramadan: Ambivalence, Fragmentation, and the Moral Self in the Lives of Young Egyptians." *Journal of the Royal Anthropological Institute* 15:S24–S40. http://www.jstor.org/stable/20527687.

———. 2012. "Surfaces of Longing Cosmopolitan Aspiration and Frustration in Egypt." *City & Society* 24 (1): 29–37. https://doi.org/10.1111/j.1548-744X.2012.01066.x.

Schneider, Marguerite. 2009. "The Difference a Word Makes: Responding to Questions on 'Disability' and 'Difficulty' in South Africa." *Disability and Rehabilitation* 31 (1): 42–50. https://doi.org/10.1080/09638280802280338.

Schwedler, J. 2010. "Amman Cosmopolitan: Spaces and Practices of Aspiration and Consumption." *Comparative Studies of South Asia, Africa and the Middle East* 30 (3): 547–562. https://doi.org/10.1215/1089201X-2010-033.

Shadid, Nasser. 2009. "جدل في الاردن حول إزالة أرحام الفتيات المعاق." BBC. July 8. https://www.bbc.com /arabic/lg/middleeast/2009/07/090708_om_jordan_mental_uterus_tc2.

Shami, Seteney. 2007. "'Amman Is Not a City': Middle Eastern Cities in Question." In *Urban Imaginaries: Locating the Modern City*, edited by Alev Cinar and Thomas Bender. University of Minnesota Press.

———. 2009. "Historical Processes of Identity Formation: Displacement, Settlement, and Self- Representations of the Circassians in Jordan." *Iran & the Caucasus* 13 (1): 141–159. http://www.jstor.org/stable/25597400.

Shaw, Alison, and Aviad Raz, eds. 2015. *Cousin Marriages: Between Tradition, Genetic Risk and Cultural Change.* 1st ed. Berghahn Books. https://www.jstor.org.aurarialibrary.idm.oclc.org/stable/j.ctt9qd0jp.

Shearer, Marsha S., and David E. Shearer. 1972. "The Portage Project: A Model for Early Childhood Education." *Exceptional Children* 39 (3): 210–217. https://doi.org/10.1177/001440297203900304.

Shryock, Andrew. 1997. *Nationalism and the Genealogical Imagination: Oral History and Textual Authority in Tribal Jordan.* University of California Press.

———. 2000. "Dynastic Modernism and Its Contradictions: Testing the Limits of Pluralism, Tribalism, and King Hussein's Example in Jordan." *Arab Studies Quarterly* 22 (3): 55–79. https://www.jstor.org/stable/41858340.

Shryock, Andrew, and Sally Howell. 2001. "'Ever a Guest in Our House': The Emir Abdullah, Shaykh Majid Al-'Adwan, and the Practice of Jordanian House Politics, as Remembered by Umm Sultan, the Widow of Majid." *International Journal of Middle East Studies* 33 (2): 247–269. https://doi.org/10.1017/S0020743801002045.

SIGI (Solidarity Is Global Institute). 2023. "تضامن تشارك في المؤتمر الختامي مع صناع القرار ضمن حملة لهنّ." December 9. https://www.sigi-jordan.org/article/6268.

Singal, Nidhi, and Nithi Muthukrishna. 2014. "Education, Childhood and Disability in Countries of the South—Re-Positioning the Debates." *Childhood* 21 (3): 293–307. https://doi.org/10.1177/0907568214529600.

Singerman, Diane. 2013. "Youth, Gender, and Dignity in the Egyptian Uprising." *Journal of Middle East Women's Studies* 9 (3): 1–27. https://doi.org/10.2979/jmiddeastwomstud.9.3.1.

Skotko, Brian. 2005. "Mothers of Children with Down Syndrome Reflect on Their Postnatal Support." *Pediatrics* 115 (1): 64–77. https://doi.org/10.1542/peds.2004-0928.

Snyder, Sharon, and David Mitchell. 2010. "Introduction: Ablenationalism and the Geo-Politics of Disability." *Journal of Literary & Cultural Disability Studies* 4 (2): 113–125. https://doi.org/10.3828/jlcds.2010.10.

Sousa, Amy C. 2011. "From Refrigerator Mothers to Warrior-Heroes: The Cultural Identity Transformation of Mothers Raising Children with Intellectual Disabilities." *Symbolic Interaction* 34 (2): 220–243. https://doi.org/10.1525/si.2011.34.2.220.

Sowt. 2024. *Eib.* https://www.sowt.com/en/podcast/eib.

Stevenson, Lisa. 2014. *Life Beside Itself: Imagining Care in the Canadian Arctic.* University of California Press.

Stiker, Henri-Jacques. 1999. *A History of Disability.* University of Michigan Press.

Strauss, Claudia. 2006. "The Imaginary." *Anthropological Theory* 6 (3): 322–344. https://doi.org/10.1177/1463499606066891.

Sukarieh, Mayssoun. 2012. "The Hope Crusades: Culturalism and Reform in the Arab World." *PoLAR: Political and Legal Anthropology Review* 35 (1): 115–134. https://doi.org/10.1111/j.1555-2934.2012.01182.x.

———. 2016. "On Class, Culture, and the Creation of the Neoliberal Subject: The Case of Jordan." *Anthropology Quarterly* 89 (4): 1201–1225. https://doi.org/10.1353/anq.2016.0073.

Summers, Ryan, Shuai Wang, Fouad Abd-El-Khalick, and Ziad Said. 2019. "Comparing Likert Scale Functionality Across Culturally and Linguistically Diverse Groups in Science Education Research: An Illustration Using Qatari Students' Responses to an Attitude Toward

Science Survey." *International Journal of Science and Mathematics Education* 17 (5): 885–903. https://doi.org/10.1007/s10763-018-9889-8.

Swedenburg, Ted. 2007. "Imagined Youths." *Middle East Research and Information Project* 245. https://merip.org/2007/12/imagined-youths/.

Sweis, Rania Kassab. 2012. "Saving Egypt's Village Girls: Humanity, Rights, and Gendered Vulnerability in a Global Youth Initiative." *Journal of Middle East Women's Studies* 8 (2): 26–50. https://doi.org/10.2979/jmiddeastwomstud.8.2.26.

Thekrallah, Fida, Ayman Qatawneh, Asma Basha, Mahmoud Al-Mustafa, Shawqi Saleh, Majed Bata, Fawaz Al-Kazaleh, and Bayan Badran. 2013. "Perceptions and Expectations Among Pregnant Women Receiving Second Trimester Ultrasound Scans at Jordan University Hospital." *Jordan Medical Journal* 47 (1): 73–79. https://doi.org/10.12816/0001071.

Thomas, Gareth M. 2017. *Down's Syndrome Screening and Reproductive Politics: Care, Choice, and Disability in the Prenatal Clinic.* Routledge.

———. 2021. "Dis-Mantling Stigma: Parenting Disabled Children in an Age of 'Neoliberal-Ableism.'" *Sociological Review* 69 (2): 451–467. https://doi.org/10.1177/0038026120963481.

———. 2024. "'We Wouldn't Change Him for the World, but We'd Change the World for Him': Parents, Disability, and the Cultivation of a Positive Imaginary." *Current Anthropology* 65 (S26). https://doi.org/10.1086/732175.

Tobin, Sarah. 2016. *Everyday Piety: Islam and Economy in Jordan.* Cornell University Press.

Tsacoyianis, Beverly A. 2021. *Disturbing Spirits: Mental Illness, Trauma, and Treatment in Modern Syria and Lebanon.* University of Notre Dame Press.

Tsing, Anna Lowenhaupt. 2005. *Friction: An Ethnography of Global Connection.* Princeton University Press.

Tucker, Judith E. 2010. *In the House of the Law: Gender and Islamic Law in Ottoman Syria and Palestine.* California University Press.

Turner, Lewis. "Who Is a Refugee in Jordan? Hierarchies and Exclusions in the Refugee Recognition Regime." *Journal of Refugee Studies* 36 (4): 877–896. https://academic.oup.com/jrs/article/36/4/877/7444737.

Turner, Victor. 1967. "Betwixt-and-Between: The Liminal Period in Rites de Passage." In *The Forest of Symbols: Aspects of Ndembu Ritual.* Cornell University Press.

———. 1969. *The Ritual Process: Structure and Anti-Structure.* 1st ed. Transaction/Routledge. https://www.routledge.com/The-Ritual-Process-Structure-and-Anti-Structure/Turner-Abrahams-Harris/p/book/9780202011905.

Twigt, Mirjam. 2022. *Mediated Lives: Waiting and Hope Among Iraqi Refugees in Jordan.* Berghahn Books.

UNHCR (United Nations High Commissioner for Refugees). 2025. "Jordan Refugee Camps." https://www.unhcr.org/jo/refugee-camps.

UNICEF. 2025. "Early Childhood Development." https://www.unicef.org/early-childhood-development.

UNICEF and MOSD (Ministry of Social Development). 2020. "دليل الإجراءات التشغيلية لبرامج التدخل المبكر في الأردن." https://www.unicef.org/jordan/media/4651/file/Standard%20Operational%20Procedures%20(SOPs).pdf.

United Nations. 2006a. *Convention on the Rights of Persons with Disabilities.* https://www.un.org/development/desa/disabilities/convention-on-the-rights-of-persons-with-Disabilities.html.

———. 2006b. اتفاقية حقوق الأشخاص ذوي الإعاقة الأمم المتحدة و البروتوكول الاختياري. https://www.un.org/disabilities/documents/convention/convoptprot-a.pdf.

UPIAS (Union of the Physically Impaired Against Segregation). 1976. "Fundamental Principles of Disability." https://disability-studies.leeds.ac.uk/wp-content/uploads/sites/40/library/UPIAS-fundamental-principles.pdf.

USAID. 2016. *Civil Society Assessment, Jordan.* https://pdf.usaid.gov/pdf_docs/PA00M5C4.pdf.

Vaidya, Shruti. 2023. "From Problem-Centered to Centering Relationalities: Engagements with Disability and Sexuality in India." *Feminist Anthropology*, September. https://doi.org/10.1002/fea2.12127.

Vinea, Ana. 2023. "Possessed or Insane? Diagnostic Puzzles in Contemporary Egypt." *International Journal of Middle East Studies* 55 (2): 260–274. https://doi.org/10.1017/S0020743823000673.

Wahlberg, Ayo, and Tine Gammeltoft. 2018. "Introduction: Kinds of Children." In *Selective Reproduction in the 21st Century*, edited by Ayo Wahlberg and Tine Gammeltoft. Palgrave Macmillan.

Washington Group. 2024. "The Washington Group on Disability Statistics." https://www.washingtongroup-disability.com/.

Watkins, Jessica. 2014. "Seeking Justice: Tribal Dispute Resolution and Societal Transformation in Jordan." *International Journal of Middle East Studies* 46 (1): 31–49. https://doi.org/10.1017/S002074381300127X.

Wehr, Hans. 1993. *The Hans-Wehr Dictionary of Modern Arabic.* 4th ed. Edited by James Cowan. Spoken Languages Services Inc. https://ejtaal.net/.

Weiss, Meira. 1994. *Conditional Love: Parents' Attitudes Toward Handicapped Children.* Bergen and Garvey.

Weldali, Maria. 2020. "HCD Prepares Procedures Manual as Special Education Facilities, Centres Reopen." *Jordan Times*, July 2. https://jordantimes.com/news/local/hcd-prepares-procedures-manual-special-education-facilities-centres-reopen.

Whitmarsh, Ian. 2008. "Biomedical Ambivalence: Asthma Diagnosis, the Pharmaceutical, and Other Contradictions in Barbados." *American Ethnologist* 35 (1): 49–63. https://doi.org/10.1111/j.1548-1425.2008.00005.x.

WHO (World Health Organization). 2022. *Global Report on Health Equity for Persons with Disabilities.* https://www.who.int/teams/noncommunicable-diseases/sensory-functions-disability-and-rehabilitation/global-report-on-health-equity-for-persons-with-disabilities.

Whyte, Susan Reynolds. 2020. "In the Long Run: Ugandans Living with Disability." *Current Anthropology* 61 (S21): S132–S40. https://doi.org/10.1086/704925.

Wikan, Unni. 1984. "Shame and Honour: A Contestable Pair." *Man* 19 (4): 635. https://doi.org/10.2307/2802330.

Willen, Sarah S. 2014. "Plotting a Moral Trajectory, Sans Papiers: Outlaw Motherhood as Inhabitable Space of Welcome." *Ethos* 42 (1): 84–100. https://doi.org/10.1111/etho.12040.

Williamson, K. Eliza. 2024. "Habilitating Bodyminds, Caring for Potential: Disability Therapeutics After Zika in Bahia, Brazil." *Cultural Anthropology* 39 (1): 9–36. https://doi.org/10.14506/ca39.1.02.

Williamson, K. Eliza, Cíntia Engel, and Helena Fietz. 2023. "The Chronicity of Home-Making: Women Caregivers in Dis/Abling Spaces." *Space and Culture* 26 (3): 468–482. https://doi.org/10.1177/12063312231181534.

Wilson, Mary Christina. 1990. *King Abdullah, Britain and the Making of Jordan.* Cambridge University Press.

Wool, Zoë H. 2021. "Disability, Straight Time, and the American Dream." *American Ethnologist* 48 (3): 288–300. https://doi.org/10.1111/amet.13027.

Wright, David. 2011. *Downs: The History of a Disability*. Oxford University Press.

Yang, Lawrence Hsin, Arthur Kleinman, Bruce G. Link, Jo C. Phelan, Sing Lee, and Byron Goode. "Culture and Stigma: Adding Moral Experience to Stigma Theory." *Social Science & Medicine* 64:1524–1535. https://doi.org/10.1016/j.socscimed.2006.11.013.

Yessayan, M. T. 2015. "Lingering in Girlhood: Dancing with Patriarchy in Jordan." *Journal of Middle East Women's Studies* 11 (1): 63–79. https://doi.org/10.1215/15525864-2832349.

Yom, Sean L. 2015. "The New Landscape of Jordanian Politics: Social Opposition, Fiscal Crisis, and the Arab Spring." *British Journal of Middle Eastern Studies* 42 (3): 284–300. https://doi.org/10.1080/13530194.2014.932271.

Zoanni, Tyler. 2019. "Appearances of Disability and Christianity in Uganda." *Cultural Anthropology* 34 (3): 444–470. https://doi.org/10.14506/ca34.3.06.

INDEX

Abdullah II, King, 117, 124n10
ableism, 19, 23, 70
abortion (termination), 45–46, 131n13, 132n14
acceptance (*taqabbul*), 2–3, 35–36, 58–59, 83;
    in affluent families, 65; making and being
    in relation to, 115–117; submission
    compared to, 77; as process, 75; question-
    ing the meaning of, 65
adab (etiquette), 68, 134n11
adolescence (*al-murahaqa*), 21, 80, 87, 94, 135n1
advocacy, 6, 7, 78, 123n2, 123n6, 131n6; cerebral
    palsy and, 30; HCD and, 32; initiatives in
    Arabic-speaking countries, 31; Jordan's
    expansion of, 80; policy change and, 35;
    toll of advocacy work, 78, 96; World Down
    Syndrome Day and, 34
aging, 19, 80, 96, 118; conflicts between
    mothers and adult children, 100; contin-
    gencies of, 113; paradoxes of, 86; of parents,
    97; as refugees, 108; social process of, 80
'ajr (merit, reward), 76, 105, 134n19, 139n20
Amman, city of, 1, 71, 82; class division in,
    9–11, *11*, *12*; dormitories for women
    migrants in, 102; Palestinian refugees in, 9,
    125n18. *See also* East Amman; West Amman
anthropology, 15, 18, 134n10; medical, 6;
    representational injustice and, 132n22
Arab Decade of Disabled Persons
    (2003–2012), 32
Arabic language, 1, 13, 17, 29, 70; switching
    between English and Arabic, 49; terms for
    Down syndrome, 30–31
assisted reproductive technologies, 46
autism spectrum disorder, 15, 30, 103, 128–129n18

al-bayt (resources of home and family), 39,
    101, 111, 117, 138n10
Bedouin, 125n20
belonging, 4, 7, 16, 39, 91
biogenetics, 47–48
biomedicine, 45, 48, 69, 85, 135n4; biomedical
    gaze, 15; husbands' authority and, 51; moral
    rubric of, 44, 59

biopolitics, 23, 47, 84, 114
biosociality, 128n17
biotechnologies, 116
blindness, 75, 128n12, 128n14
bodyminds, 2, 5, 31, 48, 60, 77; bodymind
    capacity, 78; "embodied asynchrony" as
    threat to, 19–20; genealogies of intervention
    and, 68; "normal," 20
Bourdieu, Pierre, 11

capitalism, 36
caregivers, 8–9, 18, 95
cerebral palsy, 15, 30, 75
children's rights, 84, 136n10
Christians, 10, 14, 102, 124n13, 138n12
Circassians, 13, 14, 125n20
class, 39, 55, 71, 90, 139n23; *'ayb* (shame) and,
    52; colonial/Orientalist tropes and, 27;
    difficulty in theorizing, 11; disability
    imaginaries and, 23, 64; discourse of
    "inclusion" and, 35; downward mobility,
    54; ideals of femininity and, 47; interna-
    tional division of reproductive labor and,
    7, 100; intersections with sexuality, gender,
    and age, 52; language and, 49; marital
    partnerships and, 106; marriage and, 106,
    108, 139n23; middle class, 53, 108, 137n1;
    Palestinian refugees and, 13; sartorial
    norms and, 79; working class, 10, 57, 63,
    64, 106, 137n3
consent, capacity to, 19
contraception, 85, 136n12
Council of Ifta,' 45, 92, 93
COVID-19 pandemic, 21, 32, 117–118
crip, "futures," 4; kin," 109; studies, 4; theory,
    123n4; "washing," 127n3
CRPD (U.N. Convention on Persons with
    Disabilities), 28, 29, 31, 32, 115, 128n10; HCD
    and, 90; on home and choice of residence,
    101, 102–103; human rights activism and, 74;
    on inclusive community environments, 104;
    on inclusive education, 34; Personal Status
    Law (PSL) and, 137n7; on right to marry, 105;

CRPD (cont.)
  on right to work, 110; statistics on
  hysterectomies, 91; universalizing human
  rights framework of, 100
CSOs (Civil Society Organizations), 33
culturalism, 23, 36, 40, 63, 64, 115

deafness, 75, 116, 128n12, 128n14
deinstitutionalization, 102, 103, 138n16
development, embodied, 69
diagnostic labels, "looping effects" and, 6
diagnostic technologies, prenatal, 23
disability studies, 4, 15, 18
disability: absence or eradication of, 4; as
  biopolitical category, 114; cultural meaning
  assigned to, 4; defined by CRPD, 29;
  global prevalence rate of, 27, 127n8; hidden
  by families, 22; intersections with gender
  and sexuality, 85; kinship interdependency
  and, 2, 123n3; making of, 27–34; medicalized hierarchies of, 83, 136n7; Muslims'
  understanding of, 75; proximity to, 9–11;
  reductive equation with vulnerability, 19;
  seen as "curse" or divine punishment, 57
"disability cliff," 98, 117
disability imaginaries, 16, 20, 27, 108; central
  role of hiding, 24; defined, 23, 127n2;
  developmentalist trajectory of, 115; early
  intervention and, 62; expansive, 39–40;
  shaped by culturalism, 36
disability rights, 18, 83, 93, 124n9, 127n3;
  bodily autonomy ethos and, 84, 92;
  deinstitutionalization and, 103; as "foreign"
  idea in Jordan, 28; inclusion as lynchpin of,
  24; reproductive rights and, 44; sterilization and, 90
disability worlds, 2, 28, 40, 51, 137n4
divorce, 50, 52–53, 59, 107, 125n14
Down, John Langdon, 30
Down syndrome, 1, 11, 22, 41; AMA (advanced
  maternal age) as risk factor for, 42; as
  bioethical litmus test, 5–6; causes of, 5,
  123n7, 124n8; children with Down
  syndrome as gifts from God, 54, 57, 58–59,
  74–75, 104, 134n16; health conditions
  associated with, 66, 77, 79, 133n3;
  heritability (wuratha) of, 48, 87, 136n13;
  history of, 30; language issues in description of, 30–31, 128n18; life expectancy of

people with, 5, 43, 69, 115, 119, 131n7;
  spectrum of impairment associated with,
  6; temporalities of, 2, 3–4
Down syndrome, making, 5–9, 24, 57, 124n9;
  aging and, 113; discourse of good
  motherhood and, 71; doubled discourse of
  sameness and difference, 112; kin relations
  and, 2, 3–5; kinship futures and, 116; secular
  framings of disability and, 62

early intervention (al-tadakhkhul al-
  mubakkir), 19, 22, 30, 116; advice given to
  mothers, 60; affordances and ambivalences
  associated with, 61, 66; doubled discourse
  of sameness and difference, 65–67; early
  childhood seen as critical window, 61,
  133n2; genealogies of, 67–74; imaginary of,
  63–65; interworldly, 74–77; Portage
  program, 61–62, 65, 66, 68, 133n6, 133n8;
  transitions and, 77–78
East Amman, 10, 11, 12, 16, 54, 63, 64, 65,
  71, 93
eating, challenges with, 66, 67
embodied asynchrony, 20–21, 89, 135n5;
  contested, 86–88; emplaced asynchrony
  and, 95–96; enacting of, 82–86; gendering
  of, 92–95; vital conjunctures and, 80–82
emotions, 6, 42, 71, 74, 107, 134n15
employment, 21, 110–112
endogamy, 58
English language, 17
eugenics, 84, 136n9

Facebook, 15, 31, 43, 105, 109, 118, 126n28
"family planning," 81, 85
fatwas, 45, 89, 90, 91, 92, 96, 136nn14–15
fear, as site of intervention, 72, 73, 74
feminist theory, 124n9, 132n22
fertility rates, 136n13
fetus, medicalization of, 45

Gaza, 13, 17, 61, 140n5
gender, 8, 17, 19, 108; inequalities of, 96;
  intellectual disability and, 82; intersections
  with sexuality, age, and class, 52, 81, 111;
  moral rubrics and, 56
genealogy, universal, 58
genetics, 46, 48
geopolitics, 4–5

Global North, 4, 23; debates about disability and selective reproduction, 6; focus on deinstitutionalization, 103; theorizing about disability models and politics, 33

Global South, 23, 25, 103–104

Great Arab Revolt (1916–1918), 12–13

habilitative care, 20, 61, 65, 67; early intervention and, 61

habitus, 11

Handala character, graffiti of, 82, 135n6

haraj (embarrassment), 52

Hashemites, 12, 13, 101, 129n23; civic and humanitarian leaders among, 33; "house politics" and, 39; U.S.-driven policy priorities and, 17

HCD (Higher Council for the Rights of Persons with Disabilities), 15, 27, 32, 100; COVID vaccines for disabled people and, 118; on crimes committed against disabled persons, 90; deinstitutionaliza-tion strategy and, 102; early intervention and, 133n8

heart defects, congenital, 5

heritability (*wuratha*), 46–49, 52, 55, 56

heteronormativity, 8, 96

hiding, 22, 24, 37, 38, 53; in affluent families, 65; as a core axis of disability imaginaries, 39; growth of acceptance and, 83; as human rights violation, 26; as myth and reality, 24–27

Higher Council for the Affairs of Persons with Disabilities, 33, 129n24

housing (house-ing), 21, 101–105, 113, 138n11

Humanity and Inclusion International, 36, 102

human rights, 6, 22, 25, 26, 52, 124n9

Human Rights Watch, 33, 34, 127n7

husbands, 2, 3, 22; diagnostic shock and, 43; mothers excluded from communication with doctors, 50

hypotonia (low muscle tone), 133n3

hysterectomy (removal of the uterus), 84, 85, 86, 93; CRPD statistics on, 91; families' search for doctors to perform, 90; health risks of, 136n20; menstruation removed by, 94; ruled impermissible on religious grounds, 89, 90

identity-first language, 123n1

immune system, compromised, 4, 117

"impairments" (*'ahat*), 29, 128n12; categories of, 31; early intervention and, 65, 66; of speech, 70; (*qusur*) 29

inclusion, 24, 34–38; as a core axis of disability imaginaries, 39; parents' concerns about value of education, 38–39

institutionalization, 84

intellectual disability, 75, 76, 83; culture and, 30; Down syndrome as most common genomic disorder of, 5; intersection with gender, 82; nonaccountability to recording angels, 104–105, 139n19; puberty and, 81; sterilization of women and girls with, 89

interdependencies, 8, 19, 96, 100, 103, 123n3

intersubjectivity, 86, 117

First Intifada, (1987–1993), 61, 133n5

Islam, 23, 44, 93, 134n10; global Muslim community (*ummah*), 57; Islamic bioethics, 45; Islamic inheritance law, 46; mental and legal capacity of individuals, 135n4; sartorial modesty for women, 79. *See also* Muslims; Sharia

kafala system, of labor migration, 124n11

kinship, 8, 15, 25, 123n2; "community" and, 103; contagiousness of, 48; crisis of, 44; cultural meaning assigned to Down syndrome and, 115; as diagnostic technol-ogy, 19; ethnography of, 19; family societies and, 33, 129n25; kinship terms used in Down syndrome spaces/events, 16; parenting as shared labor, 55; prenatal diagnostics and, 46

kinship futures, 2, 3–5, 18, 52, 110; aging and, 99; colonial legacies and, 12–14; constraints on, 26; diagnostic shock and, 43; effects of COVID-19 pandemic on, 117–118; embodied asynchrony and, 82, 86; gender/disability/sexuality intersection and, 85; interdependencies and, 96; making Down syndrome and, 116; marriage and, 81, 87; moral rubrics and, 59; normative trajectories of, 113; siblingship and, 21

labor markets, barriers for workers with disabilities, 39

L'arche network, 104, 138n17

Law No. 20 [Rights of Persons with Disabilities] (2017), 29, 33, 129n22, 131n5, 139n20; on definition of disability, 31; deinstitutionalization and, 102; on education of people with disabilities, 34, 133n8; embodied asynchrony and, 96; grounded in principle of antidiscrimination, 32, 137n7; HCD charter established by, 32; legality of sterilization and, 90; mirroring of CRPD, 137n7, 139n21; on right to live independently, 98, 100

marriage, 3, 4, 18, 80, 83, 97, 103, 107–108; access to, 21; boundary of adulthood marked by, 52, 87; consanguineous, 47, 58, 132n17, 132n25; demographic transitions and, 8; embodied asynchrony and, 81; heteronormative sexuality and, 4, 96; kinship futures and, 59; laws governing, 7–8, 124n12; making Down syndrome and, 51–53; marital breakdown resulting from diagnostic shock, 43, 50; marriage prospects of siblings and cousins, 42; marriage rates in Jordan, 125n15; of minors, 84; right to marry for persons with disabilities, 105–110; social regulation and, 8, 125n17
masculinity, 95, 107
masturbation, female, 136n19
masturbation, male, 92–93, 94
MENA (Middle East and North Africa), 124n10
menstruation, 83–84, 85, 86, 92, 94
mental illness, 83, 138n16
mental institutions, 127n5
Ministry of Education (MOE), 33–34, 129n22; culturalism and, 36; early intervention and, 133n8; educational reform and, 37
mongholi ("mongoloid") term, 30, 49, 57, 128n16
moral rubrics, 52–53, 56, 57, 58; interworldly, 77; kinship futures and, 59; overlapping, 44
mosaicism, 124n8
motherhood, 18, 19, 117; disability and aging, 99–101; ethnography of, 19; right to, 84
mothers, 3, 6–7, 9, 128n17; agency of, 95–96; AMA (advanced maternal age), 42; anxiety about the future, 114; blame 41, 42; as children's first trainers, 67; conflicts

with children, 19; diagnostic shock and, 43; early intervention services and, 60–62; "good" motherhood, 20, 62, 70, 71; relationships among, 70, 134n14; relations with mothers-in-law, 53–56
Muslims, 14, 54, 76, 102, 104; on living arrangements outside kinship and marriage, 102; self-cultivation among, 134n10; understanding of disability, 75; women's dress, 11; wudu' purity before prayer, 83. See also Islam; Sharia

Al-Nakba ("Catastrophe"), 13
naming practice (kunya), Arabic, 123n2
NGOs (nongovernmental organizations), 9, 23, 33
NIPT (noninvasive prenatal testing), 131n8, 131n12
nuclear family, 39, 97, 99
Al-Nur Society, 15–17, 22, 30, 34, 41, 79, 115, 118; inclusive education and, 37; outings organized by, 52; youth group of, 56

Occupied Palestine, 5, 62, 104, 118, 126n24, 133n5
Orientalism, 20, 27
ostracism, 43, 66

Palestine, mandate, 12, 13, 125n21
paraplegia, 128n12
parents: as advocates for children's pedagogical needs, 137n4; aging of, 97, 98; assumptions about future of disabled chilfren, 38; depicted as benevolent heroes, 18; diagnostic shock and, 42–44; inclusive education and, 34, 36–37; transformation of parenting over time, 99
patriarchy, 7–8, 19, 59; heritability (wuratha) and, 47, 48; legal system and, 50; "patriarchal bargain" of aging women, 109
patrilineality, 4, 7–8, 47, 59
patrilocality, 39, 101, 107
person-first language, 29, 123n1
personhood, 40, 108; affirmed through appeal to childhood, 84, 85; language and, 31, 69; nurtured in parents' home, 102
Population and Family Health Survey, 125n16, 131nn9–10

pregnancy, 55, 59, 89–90; as form of testimony, 90; medicalized and biomedicalized, 45; termination of, 115, 131n12

privacy, 19, 92

protection, right to, 89–90

puberty (*al-bulugh*), 80, 93, 135n2, 135n4; family conflict at onset of, 83; intersection with intellectual disability, 81; as traumatic rupture, 86, 94

Qur'an, 76–77, 128n14, 135n2, 139n20

race, 17

rape, 90, 91

rehabilitation, 51

rejection (*rafad*), 63, 64, 65

reproduction, 4, 7, 47, 108; "everyday biopolitics" and, 84; making Down syndrome and, 115–116; reproductive rights, 44; selective, 6

residential centers, 15, 24, 25, 50, 63, 97–98, 138n9; mothers' opposition to, 101; as negation of house-ing, 102

resource rooms, 130nn31–32

"R-word" ("r-tardation" [*takhalluf*]), 5, 123n6, 129n20, 131n6

Salamanca Statement (1994), 35

schizophrenia, 83

schooling, 4, 24, 64; inclusive education, 34–38; private schools, 34, 35, 36; public, 36, 64, 78, 125n22, 130n32

science/scientific knowledge, 56, 58, 115

sex, 85, 91, 136n19

sexual abuse, 90

sexuality, 8, 19, 47, 123n4; assumptions about men's sexuality, 92, 94; intersections with gender, age, and class, 52, 81, 85

"shadow teachers," 130n32

shame, culture of (*thaqafat al-'ayb*), 22, 83, 127n1; *'ayb* (shame), 52, 53; "honor-shame" complex, 52, 132n22

Sharia (Islamic law), 101, 107, 124n13, 138n12

shock, diagnostic, 2, 19, 42–44, 55; acceptance and, 116; dissipation of, 75; fault lines in families and, 49–51

siblings, 8, 18, 41, 53, 98; aging of, 97; care and teaching by, 95; distancing from Down syndrome siblings, 50; Down syndrome explained to, 75; hiding of disability and, 2; kinship futures and, 21; marriage prospects of, 42–43; relations of responsibility and, 78; socialization of children with Down syndrome and, 72

social media, 16, 80, 105, 126n28, 129n20; awareness campaigns on, 74; HCD and, 118

social networks, 18, 41, 53, 70

"speaking well," emphasis on, 66, 69–70

special education, 15, 16, 35, 36, 93, 103, 110; centers concentrated in Amman, 32; COVID-era closure of centers, 140n4; Ministry of Education (MOE) and, 33–34; professional training in, 39

speech therapy, 16, 69, 71

stereotypes, 30, 64, 95, 139n1

sterilization, 84, 85, 89; concealed sexual abuse and, 90; doctors in defense of, 91, 92

surveillance, technologies of, 92

SWANA (Southwest Asia and North Africa), 6, 15, 27, 124nn10–11; consanguineous marriage in, 58; efforts to eliminate marriage of minors in, 84; genealogical formulas in, 47–48; hiding of disability in, 24; historians of disability in, 29; institutionalization in, 138n16; Islamic bioethics on permissibility of abortion, 45; Portage program in, 61–62; "youth bulge" in, 80, 135n3

Syria, 5, 12, 104; civil war in, 14, 36, 108; Palestinian refugees in, 13, 125n22

tarbiyya (pedagogy), 68, 134n11

teknonyms, 1, 123n2, 134n17

time/temporalities, 61, 80; aging and temporalities of care, 98; diagnostic, 44–46; disappearance of imagined futures, 114; of kinship, 116; marriage and, 8, 106

Transjordan, Emirate of, 12–13

translocation, 123n7

"tribal" identifier, 125n20, 126n27

trisomy (triplication), in chromosome 21, 5, 34, 123n7; detectability through diagnostic technologies, 44; medical model of disability and, 50; nondisjunction as cause of, 130n2

ultrasound, second trimester, 45
United Nations (U.N.): Decade of Disabled
    Persons, 31; Statistical Commission
    City Group, 27; UNRWA (Relief and
    Works Agency), 13, 125n23. *See also*
    CRPD (U.N. Convention on Persons
    with Disabilities)
United States, 28, 79, 102; campaign against
    Islamic State, 17; "disability cliff" in, 98;
    disability prevalence rate in, 127n8;
    disability rights and awareness in, 40;
    neoliberal assaults on humanities and
    social sciences, 130n34; parents' declining
    of life-saving surgeries, 5

Vanier, Jean, 104, 138n17
violence, 7, 26, 90; curative, 4; masculinity
    and, 95; by parents, 18; postcolonial, 6;
    refugees from Iraq fleeing, 53; state-
    sponsored, 23
vital conjunctures, 80–82, 96

West, the (al-Gharb), 4, 23, 40

West Amman, 9, 10, 11, *11*, 16; access to early
    intervention services, 64
West Bank, 13, 17, 126n24
WG (Washington Group on Disability
    Statistics), 27, 28
WGSS (Washington Group Short Set), 27
WHO (World Health Organization), 27, 30, 117
Williamson, Eliza, 61
women: care labor of, 134n19; expanding
    options outside the home, 111; Islamic
    sartorial practices, 10, 11, 79; legal powers
    of male guardians, 8, 125n14; limited
    participation in labor force, 137n3; paid
    domestic workers from Africa and Asia,
    7, 124n11; property/wealth inheritance
    and, 101, 113; in public space, 10;
    responsibility for family reputation, 47.
    See also mothers
World Bank, 26
World Down Syndrome Day (March 21),
    34, 36, 105–106, 139n1

youth (*shabab*), 80, 135n1

ABOUT THE AUTHOR

CHRISTINE SARGENT is an assistant professor of anthropology at the University of Colorado, Denver. Her research interests lie at the intersections of disability, aging, kinship, and bioethics in Southwest Asia and North Africa, as well as in North America.

Available titles in the Medical Anthropology:
Health, Inequality, and Social Justice series

Carina Heckert, *Fault Lines of Care: Gender, HIV, and Global Health in Bolivia*

Joel Christian Reed, *Landscapes of Activism: Civil Society and HIV and AIDS Care in Northern Mozambique*

Alison Heller, *Fistula Politics: Birthing Injuries and the Quest for Continence in Niger*

Jessica Hardin, *Faith and the Pursuit of Health: Cardiometabolic Disorders in Samoa*

Beatriz M. Reyes-Foster, *Psychiatric Encounters: Madness and Modernity in Yucatan, Mexico*

Sonja van Wichelen, *Legitimating Life: Adoption in the Age of Globalization and Biotechnology*

Andrea Whittaker, *International Surrogacy as Disruptive Industry in Southeast Asia*

Lesley Jo Weaver, *Sugar and Tension: Diabetes and Gender in Modern India*

Ellen Block and Will McGrath, *Infected Kin: Orphan Care and AIDS in Lesotho*

Nolan Kline, *Pathogenic Policing: Immigration Enforcement and Health in the U.S. South*

Ciara Kierans, *Chronic Failures: Kidneys, Regimes of Care, and the Mexican State*

Stéphanie Larchanché, *Cultural Anxieties: Managing Migrant Suffering in France*

Dvera I. Saxton, *The Devil's Fruit: Farmworkers, Health, and Environmental Justice*

Siri Suh, *Dying to Count: Post-Abortion Care and Global Reproductive Health Politics in Senegal*

Vania Smith-Oka, *Becoming Gods: Medical Training in Mexican Hospitals*

Daria Trentini, *At Ansha's: Life in the Spirit Mosque of a Healer in Mozambique*

Mette N. Svendsen, *Near Human: Border Zones of Species, Life, and Belonging*

Cristina A. Pop, *The Cancer Within: Reproduction, Cultural Transformation, and Health Care in Romania*

Elizabeth J. Pfeiffer, *Viral Frictions: Global Health and the Persistence of HIV Stigma in Kenya*

Anna Versfeld, *Making Uncertainty: Tuberculosis, Substance Use, and Pathways to Health in South Africa*

Tanja Ahlin, *Calling Family: Digital Technologies and the Making of Transnational Care Collectives*

Sarah A. Smith, *Forgotten Bodies: Imperialism, Chuukese Migration, and Stratified Reproduction in Guam*

Danya Fast, *The Best Place: Addiction, Intervention, and Living and Dying Young in Vancouver*

Michelle Pentecost, *The Politics of Potential: Global Health and Gendered Futures in South Africa*

Mirko Pasquini, *The Negotiation of Urgency: Economies of Attention in an Italian Emergency Room*

Lily N. Shapiro, *Connective Tissue: Factory Accidents and Reconstructive Plastic Surgery in South India*

Christine Sargent, *Making Down Syndrome: Motherhood and Kinship Futures in Urban Jordan*